Military Retirement: Social, Economic, and Mental Health Dilemmas

In 1940 there were 48,000 military retirees; today there are well over a million. This book is the first critical, objective study of the difference between "normal" retirement and military retirement, and its impact on retirees, their families, and society in general. Beginning with an historical overview, the authors examine how the often short-sighted policies of the American military have led to social, economic, and mental health problems of enormous proportions, and conclude with an analysis of current trends and their implications for the future.

Military Retirement: Social, Economic, and Mental Health Dilemmas

John S. McNeil
Associate Professor, Graduate School of Social Work, The University of Texas at Arlington. Colonel, United States Air Force, Retired

Pedro J. Lecca
Professor, Graduate School of Social Work, The University of Texas at Arlington. Lt. Colonel, Army Reserve

Roosevelt Wright, Jr.
Associate Professor
Graduate School of Social Work, The University of Texas at Arlington.

Rowman & Allanheld
PUBLISHERS

ROWMAN & ALLANHELD

Published in the United States of America in 1983
by Rowman & Allanheld
(A division of Littlefield, Adams & Company)
81 Adams Drive, Totowa, New Jersey 07512

Library of Congress Cataloging in Publication Data

McNeil, John S., 1927–
Military retirement.

Bibliography: p.
Includes index.
1. United States—Armed Forces—Appointments and
retirements—Addresses, essays, lectures. I. Lecca,
Pedro J., 1936– . II. Wright, Roosevelt.
III. Title.
UB323.M36 1983 305'.90697'0973 83-3281
ISBN 0-86598-078-0

83 84 85/ 10 9 8 7 6 5 4 3 2 1

Printed in the United States of America

Dedicated to

My wife, Bettye B. McNeil

My mother and father, the Pedro J. Lecca, Srs., and Uncles Francisco, Eugene, y Sanchez.

My mother and father, Roosevelt and Ruth Wright.

CONTENTS

LIST OF TABLES AND FIGURES

TABLES

FIGURES

PREFACE

Since its inception in 1861, military retirement has retained its basic structure. Permeating the history of military retirement, however, has been an attempt to determine the degree of physical stamina and mental acumen necessary for the performance of military duty at a satisfactory level. It was not until World War II that military manpower policy specifically addressed a youth and vigor concept. Undoubtedly this concern was epitomized in the establishment of the twenty-year retirement authorization as permanent policy following World War II. Youth and vigor were not clearly defined in operational terms and there was lack of attention to the need for an across the board policy that included all job categories or whether it should apply only to certain specialized functions. This issue was raised specifically by the President's Commission on Military Compensation that was empaneled in 1976. Members of the commission asked four questions in their quest for information that would assist in policy making. These questions were:

1. What elements within the armed forces appear to have a genuine need for youth and vigor?
2. What findings are provided in the technical literature concerning loss of performance capability, and loss of specific human capacities, as a function of chronological age, up to age sixty?

3. Are there reasonable methods that could be used to quantify youth and vigor, other than chronological age?
4. Will appropriate training and conditioning techniques help to maintain adequate youth and vigor in military personnel over age forty? (Parker, et al., 1978)

It is readily apparent that these questions strike at the core of the isssue of allowing retirement eligibility to be attained by individuals who are in their late thirties or early forties. Challenged was the justification that all military personnel must be prepared at all times to go into combat under the most rigorous of conditions. Relative to question number one, Parker and his cohorts concluded that an excellent case could be made in certain very specialized units (it was estimated 12 percent of enlisted personnel are in combat assignments) but that the majority of individuals are in support functions that do not require youth and vigor (Parker, et al., 1978).

Parker and his associates reviewed numerous studies that attempted to demonstrate the effects of age on human capacities. They examined data regarding physical activities, physiological function, sensory functions, perceptual-motor processes, mental processes, and the effects of selection, training, and conditioning. These findings were then weighed against work performance. Additionally, attempts have been made to develop an index of "functional age," but these efforts have met with little success. Except for combat-type units Parker and his cohorts concluded that no concrete argument could be offered to justify a youthful and vigorous military force of individuals with an average age in their twenties. Further it was suggested that sound judgment, which grows out of experience, may be more crucial than youth and vigor. Parker also pointed out that age does have some effect upon human capacities, but significant age-deficits are not found until the sixth or seventh decades of life. Some exceptions may be found in tasks that require superior visual acuity, strength, or rapid reaction time. Finally, attempts to develop an index of "functional age" have for the most part met with failure (Parker, et al., 1978).

Youth and vigor has not been defined satisfactorily to date. Operationally, however, it appears to refer to the performance of individuals between the ages of forty and sixty years. Implementing a policy of youth and vigor therefore necessitates maintaining a military force of personnel with a relatively low average age. The average age of active duty enlisted personnel is age twenty-five and is approximately thirty-three years for officers (Holmes, et al., 1978). In fiscal year 1981 the average age of officers who retired was forty-five and for enlisted personnel the average age at retirement was forty (Defense Manpower Data Center, 1981). A policy embracing the youth and vigor concept therefore influences the entire military personnel management process. In order to maintain a military force with an average age of approximately twenty-nine or thirty the top age of entry must be controlled and there must be mechanisms for voluntary or involuntary removal of individuals from active military service while they are relatively young. As a result the military recruits late adolescents and young adults primarily and has developed policies that encourage individuals to leave the uniformed services at an early age. These values are reflected in much of the retirement legislation and regulations. The following table itemizes some descriptions of youth and vigor and the values appearing in legislation.

Description	Values appearing in legislation
Maximum age to remain on active duty	50, 60, 62, 64
Age vs. grade	O-7, 64; O-6, 56; O-5, 50; O-1 to O-4, 45
Years of service vs. grade	O-8, 35; O-7 and O-6, 30; O-5, 28; O-4, 21 or 20; O-3, 14; O-2, 7
Length of service	45, 40, 30, 10, 16, 15
Non-selection for promotion	Twice fail
Involuntary released from active duty	Inefficient, poor potential; retired if over 7, 10, 20 years of service; otherwise severance pay

Source: Holmes, et al., 1978

Years of service exit points are usually reached before age points of exit. In order to remain on active duty for more than thirty years the individual must have attained the rank of two star general, which is highly unlikely for most military members. Values reflected in retirement legislation indicate a decided leaning in the direction of a youthful and vigorous military force.

A central focus of this book will be to review and evaluate the impact of youth and vigor as it relates to the military retirement program. The development of this concept will be traced in the chaper on the history of military retirement. The social, economic, and mental health implications will be discussed in subsequent chapters.

J.S.M.
P.J.L.
R.W., Jr.

1

HISTORY OF MILITARY RETIREMENT

Introduction

Military retirement history may be seen as having three overlapping but fairly distinct phases. The first phase would encompass the period from colonization to the Civil War. The second period extends from the Civil War to World War II. The third phase is from World War II to the present. Retirement eligibility determined solely on the basis of battle-connected injury characterized the initial period. Following this was a period when military retirement eligibility could be obtained on the basis of age and/or length of service. Attention was also given to the idea of physical fitness to perform military duty. This latter concern led to a major characterization of the present phase, an emphasis upon youth and vigor, which has resulted in the earlier-retirement eligibility criteria that has led to an almost geometric increase in the size of the military retired rolls. These three phases in the history of military retirement will be discussed separately, beginning with the span of time from colonial days to the Civil War.

The Colonial Period to the Civil War

Members of the military services have received special legislative attention since colonial days. As early as 1636, Plymouth Colony legislated that any man who performed duty as a soldier and returned from battle totally disabled should be maintained by the Colony. In 1661, the General Assembly of Maryland ruled:

> Every person that shall adventure as a Souldier in any warre in the defence of the Country and shall therein happen to be maymed or receive hurt, shall according to his place and Quality receive mayntenance from the Country according to his disability for mayntayning him selfe. (U.S. Congress, Committee on Veterans' Affairs, 1955).

Virginia passed similar legislation in 1675 and Rhode Island did likewise in 1718. (Committee on Veterans' Affairs, 1955).

Prior to the emergence of the colonies into a national government, each colony assumed responsibility for its disabled servicemen. Most of this legislation was essentially similar in that it was premised upon battle-connected disability and impairment must have been suffered to such an extent that the individual was unable or partially unable to earn a living.

This precedent was followed by the Continental Congress and in August 1776 the federal government undertook responsibility for disabled servicemen. Spurred by the Revolutionary War then in progress, the Continental Congress appointed a "committee on disabled soldiers and seamen" to study the problem. Eventually Congress agreed on the following provisions:

> Whereas in the course of the present war, some commissioned and non-commissioned officers as also private soldiers, marines and seamen, may lose a limb, or be otherwise so disabled as to prevent their serving in the army, or navy or getting livelihood, and may stand in the need of relief:
>
> Resolved, That every commissioned officer, non-commissioned officer, and private soldier, who shall lose a limb in any

> engagement, or be so disabled in the service of the United States of America as to render him incapable afterwards of getting a livelihood, shall receive, during his life, or the continuance of such disability, the one half of his monthly pay from and after the time his pay as an officer or soldier ceases; to be paid by the committee as hereafter mentioned.
>
> That every commissioned officer, non-commissioned officer and private soldier, in the army . . . who shall be wounded in any engagement, so as to be rendered incapable of serving in the army . . . though not totally disabled from getting a livelihood, shall receive such monthly sum towards his subsistence as shall be judged adequate by the assembly or other respresentative body of the state where he belongs or resides, upon application to them for that purpose, provided the same doth not exceed his half pay. (*U.S. Air Force News for Retired Personnel,* April 1961)

The First Congress of the United States thus continued the precedent of providing pensions for those veterans who were totally or partially disabled. In the case of partial disability, however, it appears payment was to be made by the federal government, but the amount of pension to be paid was determined locally.

Another precedent was established in 1818 when Revolutionary War veterans who had not been disabled in battle were eligible for pensions if they were in need of assistance. Even though an income test was required, the act laid the groundwork for pensions to veterans of subsequent wars during their later years of life. The so-called "pauper clause" inserted into the 1818 law came up for review when the act was amended in 1832. Representative Henry Hubbard of New Hampshire adamantly fought against the clause during the House debate. He argued in vain that "many, very many, even at this day [obviously referring to the advanced ages of Revolutionary veterans in 1832] chose to forego the benefits of the pension system than to make the humiliating, the mortifying declaration of abject poverty . . ." (Committee on Veterans' Affairs, 1955). The majority argued that individuals worth as much as "five thousand dollars" could collect the pension if an income test were not required.

No significant change was made in military pension provisions until 1861, although during the intervening years pension legislation had been passed dealing with each war, including the numerous Indian skirmishes. It should also be mentioned that benefits were usually available for surviving dependents if the serviceman was killed during battle. Of particular import regarding these earlier programs is that they provided only for disability pensions and there was no provision for retirement on the basis of age or years of military service. No system, therefore, was available to remove superannuated individuals from the military service active duty rolls. This stagnating situation was dramatized as preparations for the Civil War commenced.

The Civil War to World War II

The second phase in the history of military retirement began during the Civil War and lasted until about the Second World War. During this period nondisability retirement was authorized through Congressional legislation. In 1855, however, provisions were enacted for Navy officers to be retired for reasons other than physical disability if they were found to be incapable of performing duty. Mobilization for the Civil War necessitated a much broader based retirement authority that would include the Army, Navy, and Marine Corps.

The need for a retirement system was recognized for many years by military personnel planners, but because no legislation authorized retirement, personnel could hang on literally until death regardless of their ability to perform military duty. A prime example occurred during the Mexican War (1846–1848); only a limited number of senior officers had been authorized in the regular army and one of these positions was held tenaciously by a "senile octogenarian," a Colonel Walback. One Army historian wrote that at the beginning of the Civil War, practically all field grade officers in the Army (i.e., all officers above the grade of captain) were physically incapable of exercising command in the field (Ganoe, 1942). Further evidence of the need for retirement legislation may be found in the following quote: "When the Civil War started the junior Captain in the U.S. Navy had 42 years of service, and the average Captain in the Army was in his fifties. Many of the Majors in the Army were in their sixties and seventies. In fact the commanding officer of the Army at that time was General Winfield Scott, who was 82 years old and 325 pounds and used a block and tackle to get up on his horse" (Parker, Christensen, and Every, 1978).

These examples planted the seeds for later emphasis upon the need for a military force composed of youthful and vigorous individuals. Until well into the twentieth century, management of military forces relied upon normal attrition (i.e., death and disability) for personnel turnover and as could be expected proved ineffective. The concepts of youth and vigor are critical issues in military retirement planning at this time and many points of view are heatedly debated regarding their definition and implementation. In 1860, however, youth and vigor were only seminal ideas.

On July 14, 1861, President Lincoln signed the General Law Pension System Bill, which went into effect at the beginning of the following year. This bill provided for a military retirement program for those officers with "long and faithful service." Additionally, it continued the disability pension system. No specific action was taken regarding retirement for enlisted personnel, except in the case of a service-connected disability. Among the more important provisions of the 1861 act were the following:

1. It provided for voluntary retirement of officers after forty years of service.
2. It provided for involuntary retirement of officers with forty-five years of service, at Presidential discretion.
3. It provided for disability retirement of disabled servicemen (enlisted personnel were included here).
4. It provided for retirement pay computed on the basis of military rank (U.S. Congress, 1861).

This law, it can be seen, was primarily a personnel management tool, in contrast to the humanitarian features of previous disability pension legislation. The basic framework of this law has remained in effect up to the present. Of particular importance in the 1861 act is that the noncontributory principle utilized in service-connected disability pensions was continued. It should be pointed out, however, that military retirement was the first retirement program initiated in America. The first retirement program in private industry did not begin until more than a decade later. Also of interest is that retired pay continued to be based upon previous earnings (prior military rank).

Almost twenty-five years later, 1885, enlisted men became eligible for nondisability retirement if they had at least thirty years of military service (U.S. Congress, *Statutes At Large*, Forty-seventh Congress, First Session, Ch. 254, 1882). In 1892 disability pensions were authorized for female nurses who had served in the Civil War (Title 27, U.S. Statute 348, 1892). It was 1926 before nondisability retirement was authorized for nurses (Title 44, U.S. Statute 531, 1926).

Between the Civil War and the turn of the century, some feeble attempts were made to control the size of the military retired rolls. These efforts did not deal with the youth and vigor concepts nor did they provide military managers with an effective personnel control mechanism. The Army limited the size of the retired rolls to 400, but this procedure in effect forced superannuated individuals to remain on active duty. The Navy did not allow retirement until the officer reached the age of sixty-two. Similar to the Army, the Navy policies encouraged individuals to remain on active duty until their ability to perform effectively could be questioned (Parker, Christensen, and Every, 1978).

In 1870 the Navy introduced a significant policy, recomputation. A decision was made that a balance should be maintained between active duty pay and retired pay. Whenever military active duty pay was increased, retired pay was recomputed on the basis of the active duty pay raise. If an individual was retired after having served thirty years of military duty, for example, his retired pay would be recomputed as if he was just retiring when an active duty pay raise was enacted. This procedure was followed by all branches of military service until 1958, when a change was made to adjust retired pay in accordance with the cost of living index. As will be discussed later, this change was seen as a breach of faith against an implied right and an institutionalized entitlement. Recomputation dealt strictly with periodic increases in retired pay, but the basic structure of the General Law Pension System bill remained intact.

Although the framework of the bill remained the same, three factors had been manipulated that impacted upon implementation of retirement actions. These factors were: 1. number of years required to attain retirement eligibility, 2. advancement in grade at the time of retirement, and 3. the formula utilized to determine the amount of retired pay the retiree would receive.

The number of years required to attain retirement eligibility has varied from a high of forty-five to as few as seven under special circumstances. The number of years have also varied according to whether or not the retirement was voluntary or involuntary. In general the trend has been toward requiring fewer years in order to be eligible for retirement. Voluntary retirement initially (1861) required forty years; in 1870 this was reduced to thirty years and at present twenty years is required to attain eligibility. Interspersed with these decreases have been periods of time that personnel could retire with even fewer years when it was necessary to meet special force reduction needs. During World War I, the Navy and Marine Corps placed individuals in the Fleet Naval Reserve with sixteen years service. This had the effect of retirement. In 1920, the Army allowed for retirement of "Class B" officers who had over ten years of active duty. In 1935, the Army, Navy, and Marine Corps authorized retirement with less than twenty years service. The Army permitted retirement for officers after fifteen years if they had served as Philippine Scouts, apparently referring to individuals who had been on active duty during the Spanish American War (U.S. Congress, 1935). The Navy, in 1935, began authorizing the retirement of lieutenants with fourteen years service and lieutenants, junior grade with seven years service. Both of these measures appear to have been prompted by a concern for youth and vigor, to meet force reduction needs, and as a means of quality control. It seems that twenty years of service was eventually arrived at as the modal figure to attain minimum retirement eligibility.

Military rank is another factor that has been manipulated relative to retirement. On various occasions, military officers have been promoted to the next higher grade upon retirement with or without receiving the pay of the elevated grade. In 1899, legislation was enacted that allowed the Navy to involuntarily retire "up to five Captains, four Commanders, four Lieutenant Commanders and two Lieutenants each year . . . to create necessary vacancies." These mandatorily retired officers were to receive three-quarters of the sea pay of the next higher grade. Within a few years all branches of the military authorized promotion upon retirement and receipt of the pay of the next higher grade (Title 30, U.S. Statute 1006, 1899). Such action was for a special group of officers only, but for a different reason than the 1899 act. The earlier provision would appear to have been a means of compensation to decrease the stigma of involuntary retirement. The latter act was reserved for officers "who had served with credit during the Civil War." Here, the promotion seems to be an attempt to stimulate the retirement of elderly officers. Promotions have been authorized at retirement at other times, but the individuals did not receive the pay of the next higher rank. An example of this was the so-called "tombstone promotion" of Navy officers that occurred during the 1920s.

Retired pay throughout the years of the history of disability and nondisability retirement has been computed on the basis of 50 or 75 percent of the service person's active duty pay. Since 1916, the amount of retired pay began to be determined on the basis of 2.5 percent of active duty pay multiplied by the number of years of service, but not to exceed 75 percent of active duty pay. While this has been the standard formula for the computation of the amount of retired pay, variations have occurred. When the Navy authorized retirement after sixteen years of service in 1916, the retiree received one-third of active duty pay. Following World War I, involuntarily retired Army officers with over twenty years of military service received three percent of their active duty pay multiplied by the number of years service, not to exceed 75 percent of their active duty pay. This same legislation limited warrant officers under certain circumstances to two percent of active duty pay multiplied by number of years of service.

Manipulation of two of these factors—years of service needed to attain full retirement eligibility and the formula for determining the amount of retired pay to which a recipient would be entitled—have been included in some of the current proposals to overhaul the military retirement program. Considerable pressure has been exerted to change the military retirement program, primarily to reduce the rapidly escalating costs. Countering this effort to control the cost has been the emphasis upon youth and vigor. This policy has tended to necessitate retirement at a relatively young age therefore increasing the size of the retirement rolls and increasing retirement costs. World War II witnessed the beginning of a new historical phase regarding military retirement with special attention being given to manpower policies and costs.

World War II to the Present

Policies were established during and immediately after World War II that entrenched the twenty-year retirement system. In 1945, voluntary retirement of Army enlisted personnel was authorized after twenty years of active duty and this privilege was extended to Navy and Marine officers if they had at least ten years of commissioned service. Similar provisions were enacted for Army officers in 1948. With the establishment of the Air Force, all Army retirement policies were made applicable for the new branch of service. Within two years after the end of World War II, all branches of the military service authorized retirement after twenty years of active duty for officers and enlisted personnel. The twenty-year retirement authority was embodied in the Army and Air Force Vitalization and Retirement Equalization Act of 1948 (Title 62, U.S. Statute 1081, 1948).

Retirement after twenty years service was not a unanimous decision. A Department of Defense Advisory Commission on Service Pay headed by Charles R. Hook recommended an increase in the time required for retirement eligibility (Hook, 1948). The Hook Commission suggested that officers be permitted to retire after thirty years of service or at age sixty with twenty years of service. Enlisted personnel should be authorized retirement after twenty-five years service or at age fifty with twenty years of service. The Army supported the Hook proposals as being sound and equitable and would not have long-run negative effects. The Air Force and Navy were against the thirty-year retirement recommendation and argued that it would stifle promotions, effect transfer of members to the Reserves, and impede the recruitment and retention of younger enlisted personnel (*Report of President's Commission on Military Compensation*, 1978).

The Navy and Air Force arguments prevailed, therefore reinforcing the youth and vigor concept. Another factor was also at work, which was the realization that a relatively large-sized active duty force would be required for some period of time. To enhance its effectiveness, an efficient Reserve force was needed, and to facilitate its establishment a retirement system was authorized in 1948 for the military reserves and the National Guard as an incentive to hold personnel for longer periods of time. Career Reservists may qualify for retired pay after twenty years of satisfactory service. Retired pay, however, cannot be drawn until the individual is age sixty and at that time he and his dependents are eligible for all benefits that accrue to personnel who retired from the regular military forces.

Another important statute that was enacted after World War II was the Officer Personnel Act of 1947, which inaugurated the "up or out" policy. Officers of designated grades who failed to be promoted by the time they attained specified years of service were involuntarily retired or released from

Table 1.1 Summary of Officer Personnel Act of 1947

Pay grade	Army and Air Force	Navy and Marine Corps
O–10, O–9[a]	Retired after 5 years in grade or 35 years of service, but retirement may be deferred to age 64.	Retired after 5 years in grade and 35 years of service, unless selected for continuation.
O–8	Retired after 5 years in grade or 35 years of service, but retirement may be deferred to age 60.	Retired after 5 years in grade and 35 years of service, unless selected for continuation.
O–7	Retired after 5 years in grade or 30 years of service, but retirement may be deferred to age 60.	Rear Admiral (lower half) retired after 5 years in grade and 35 years of service unless selected for continuation; Brigadier General, USMC-Retired after second failure of selection for promotion.
O–6	Retired after 5 years in grade or 30 years of service.	Retired after 30 years in service if twice failed of selection for promotion, or after 31 years if not twice failed.
O–5	Retired after 28 years of service.	Retired after 26 years of service if twice failed of selection for promotion.
O–4, O–3 O–2, O–1	When twice passed over for promotion: Retired if have 20 years of service; retained to complete 20 years and then retired if within 2 years of 20-year point; eliminated with severance pay if less than 18 years of service.	O–4 retired after 20 years of service if twice failed of selection for promotion; other grades eliminated with severance pay if twice failed.

[a]Officer ranks range from O–1 to a high of O–10.
Source: Third Quadrennial Review of Military Compensation, 1978

Table 1.2 Involuntary Nondisability Retirement Provisions for Officers

Year	Provisions
1855	Nonphysical disability (Navy)
1861	45 years of service (YOS)[a] *or* 62 years of age (YOA)[a], Service Secretary Discretion (Navy)
1862	Army/Marine Corps; same as 1861 Navy
1873	45 YOS *and* 62 YOA, Service Secretary Discretion
1882	64 YOA (Army)
1890	Twice fail promotion, severance pay (Army)
1899	Specified number of O–3 to O–6's[b] if not enough voluntary retirements (Navy)
1916	Nonselected O–6, 56 YOA; O–5, 50 YOA; O–4, 45 YOA: any grade, 65 YOA (Navy)
1920	Class "B" officers retired if over 10 YOS, discharged with severance pay if under 10 YOS (Army)
1922	Reduction in commissioned strength, under 10 YOS discharged with severance pay, over 10 YOS retired (Army); non-Naval Academy officers exempt from age vs. grade limits (O–4 to O–6), completion of specified time in grade required (Navy)
1925	If fail promotion: under 10 YOS, discharged with severance pay; over 10 YOS, retired as follows: O–6, 56 YOA; O–5, 50 YOA, O–1 to O–4, 45 YOA (Marine Corps)
1926	Navy age/grade changed to YOS/grade: O–6, 35 YOS; O–5, 28 YOS, O–4, 21 YOS (Navy)

active duty with a lump sum payment if they had not attained retirement eligibility. The essential provisions of this act are shown in Table 1.1.

Although the statutory "up or out" policy was in force, it was not sufficient to remove the excess of senior officers who remained on active duty as a result of the peak buildup of forces during World War II. Therefore, the Navy in 1959 and the Army and Air Force in 1960 enacted procedures for the mandatory retirement of officers in pay grades O-5 and O-6 before they reached the twenty-six, twenty-eight, or thirty years of service phase points. Those officers selected for

Table 1.2, cont.

1931	O–3's, 45 YOA *and* 20 YOS, if fail promotion exam (Navy)
1934	Marine Corps provisions same as Navy
1935	O–2, 14 YOS; O–3, 21 YOS (Navy/Marine Corps)
1936	O–4, 21 YOS; O–5, 28 YOS; if not on promotion list (Marine Corps)
1938	Promotion by selection rather than age or service in grade. O–2 to O–4: if fail selection twice, retired (over 20 YOS), discharged with severance pay (under 20 YOS); O–5, O–6: if fail selection twice, retired (Navy/Marine Corps)
1941	Army Vitalization Act. Inefficient officers discharged (under 7 YOS), retired (over 7 YOS) (Army)
1947	Officer Personnel Act. Army/Air Force: Major General, 62 YOA. All other 60 YOA *or* not selected for promotion and: O–8, 35 YOS or 5 years in grade; O–5, 28 YOS; O–4, 21 YOS; O–3, 14 YOS (severance pay); O–2, 7 YOS (severance pay). Navy/Marine Corps: O–7, not recommended for continuation after twice considered. All others, twice fail selection and O–6, 30 YOS: O–5, 26 YOS; O–4, 20 YOS; O–3, O–2, severance pay.
1948	Show cause board, retired if over 15 YOS, otherwise discharged with severance pay
1959	O–4, O–5 with least potential, retired early (Navy/Marine Corps)
1960	O–5, O–6 not reaching expected potential, retired early (Army/Air Force)

[a]YOS means Years of Service and YOA means Years of Age.
[b]Officer rank ranges from a low of O–1 to a high of O–10.
Source: Holmes, R.A., et al., 1978.

involuntary retirement were considered to be noncompetitive with their contemporaries. Being labeled substandard, however, angered many of the affected officers and the action was challenged in court, but to no avail. Involuntary retirement has been used as a manpower management tool since the beginning of the nondisability retirement system. Legislation has typically applied only to officers. Table 1.2 presents a chronology of the consistency with which involuntary retirement has been utilized for over a hundred years.

There have been no significant changes in the military retirement personnel procedures since the Army and Air Force

Vitalization and Retirement Equalization Act of 1948. Change in this instance speaks specifically at personnel measures and does not include the 1958 policy that discontinued recomputation as a means of adjusting retired pay and shifted instead to the Consumer Price Index. Between 1948 and 1979 several major studies of military compensation, including retirement were made. Among these were the Hook Commission study (Hook, 1948), two of the three Quadrennial Reviews of Military Compensation (Quadrennial Review of Military Compensation: First, 1969; and Third, 1977), the Interagency Committee study (Interagency Committee, 1971), and the Defense Manpower Commission study (Defense Manpower Commission, 1976). Each of these studies have recommended considerable change in the current military retirement system. For the most part these recommendations have encouraged extending the number of years required to attain full retirement eligibility. Additionally, attention has been given as to whether or not there should be some vesting privilege and/or alternative system of compensation for individuals who leave the military service prior to attaining minimum retirement eligibility. Currently, personnel who elect to leave the uniformed services before having served twenty years are not eligible for any retirement benefits and have no withdrawal or vesting rights.

Robert Hale of the Congressional Budget Office has compared several of the proposals with the present system while holding constant the point in time that the retirement annuity becomes payable. Hale's table is reproduced as Table 1.3.

It can be seen that several substantive changes have been recommended. Provisions would be made for the vesting of retired pay if the individual had been on active duty for more than ten years but less than twenty years. The amount of the retired pay would be related to both age and years of service. Reduced annuities would be paid to individuals who had served less than thirty years of active duty dependent upon the age of the retiree. Upon attainment of age levels between fifty-five and sixty, the annuity would be increased. Lump sum payments would be made to both enlisted and officer personnel who were involuntarily released from active duty with over

Table 1.3 Detailed Provisions of Alternative Retirement Systems

	Current system	Reduced annuity to 30 years of service	Reduced annuity to age 55 or 60	Annuity to Age 55 to 62
Retirement Base	Terminal basic pay.	High-1 basic pay.	High-3 basic pay.	High-3 basic pay.
Formula for Computing Annuity (Voluntary Separation)	Retirement base times 2.5 percent per YOS (maximum 75 percent.	Retirement base times 2.5 percent per YOS (10–24 YOS) plus 3 percent per YOS (25–30 YOS) to maximum of 78 percent, less 15 percentage points until time when 30 YOS would have been completed.	Retirement base times 2.5 percent per YOS (10–24 YOS) plus 2 percent per YOS (31–35 YOS) to maximum of 88 percent. Annuity reduced until age 60 (less than 25 YOS) or age 55 (25 or more YOS). Reduction equals 2 percent of annuity for each year under age threshold.	Retirement base times 2.5 percent per YOS (maximum 87.5 percent).
When Annuity Begins (Voluntary Separation)	More than 20 YOS: upon retirement; 0–19 YOS: no benefits.	More than 20 YOS: upon retirement; 10–19 YOS: age 60[a]; 0–9 YOS: no benefits.	More than 20 YOS: upon retirement (with reduction if applicable); 10–19 YOS: lump-sum payment equal to 5 percent YOS times terminal basic pay[b]; 0–9 YOS: no benefits.	More than 30 YOS: age 55; 20–29 YOS: age ___; 5–19 YOS: age 62; 0–4 YOS: no benefits.
Formula for Computing Annuity (Involuntary Separation)	Entlisted: no annuity[c]; officer: lump-sum payment equal to 10 percent times	More than 20 YOS: same as voluntary; 5–19 YOS: lump-sum payment of	More than 20 YOS: same as voluntary; plus lump-sum payment equal	More than 5 YOS: same as voluntary plus lump-sum payment equal to percent

Table 1.3, cont.

	YOS times retirement base (maximum $15,000).	10 percent times YOS times terminal basic pay[b]; 0–4 YOS: no benefits.	to 5 percent per YOS times terminal basic pay; 5–9 YOS: lump-sum payment equal to 5 percent per YOS times terminal basic pay; 0–4 YOS: no benefits.	per YOS times terminal basic pay; 0–4 YOS: no benefits.
Social Security Integration	None	Annuity reduced by half of social security payments attributable to military service.	Annuity reduced by half of social security payments attributable to military service.	None
Reduction for Continued Federal Employment (Double Dipping)	Over 20 YOS: regular officers forfeit about 1/3 of annuity.	Same as current system.	Same as current system.	Same as current system.
Price Adjustment	Automatic based on CPI.	Same as current system[d]	Same as current system.	Same as current system.
Phase-In Period for Reduced Annuities for Early Retirees	Not Applicable	20 years	10 years	10 years
Save-Pay Provisions	Not applicable	Individualized[e]	Individualized[e]	None

Note: YOS = Years of Service.

[a]If retiree dies before the deferred annuity starts, survivors receive a lump-sum payment.

[b]Retirees have a choice of a lump sum or deferred annuity. In this paper, all are assumed to elect the lump sum.

[c]Enlisted receive involuntary separation pay in a few circumstances, but these are ignored in this paper.

[d]Deferred annuities are adjusted for price increases between retirement and the time when payment begins.

[e]Individualized save-pay insures that a retiree's pay would be at least as much as it would have been if, at some year, he had been eligible and had chosen to retire.

Source: Hale, 1978.

five years of active duty but less than twenty years. Several benefits are expected to accrue from these recommended changes: 1. They would encourage career individuals to remain on active duty for longer periods of time, 2. They would also encourage noncareer personnel to vest their retirement and leave the military service when fewer people are needed at middle management levels, and 3. They would facilitate manpower management by offering a more humane involuntary separation mechanism.

Not mentioned in these proposals, however, is the issue of a contributory vs. a noncontributory retirement funding system. All of the studies except one have recommended continuation of the present noncontributory system (issues regarding funding are discussed in Chapter 2).

In view of the persistent and intense interest evidenced toward the military retirement system over the past three decades, the likelihood is quite high that some significant changes will be made in the future. These changes will more than likely alter the early retirement privilege based upon the youth and vigor concept.

2

ECONOMIC DILEMMAS OF MILITARY RETIREMENT

Introduction

The economics of the military retirement system may be evaluated relative to its impact upon the individual retiree, the military establishment, and the national economy. This chapter is not intended to be an economic treatise of military retirement; rather several important aspects will be described and discussed. The controversial and complicated nature of many of the issues will be highlighted. Specific attention will be given to the nondisability and disability retirement programs, survivor benefits, the relationship of the military retirement program with social security, restrictive legislation, and the unfunded liability issue.

Size of Rolls and Costs

Military retirement attracted relatively little public attention until approximately twenty years ago. Although congressional legislation was enacted during the Civil War that authorized the establishment of a military retirement system, no comprehensive study was made of it until after World War II. This study, which was done by the Hook Commission, evaluated several aspects of the program such as benefits, eligibility for benefits, and funding. A few years later in 1953, the first actuarial evaluation of the program was completed. The retirement program, therefore, had been in operation for over ninety years before an intensive review of its cost was made. Since 1960, several major studies have been done of the military retirement program. The impetus for this dramatic increase in attention has been related directly to the cost factor and its twin, the number of people on the retired roll. Prior to World War II the size of the military retired rolls was reasonably small and consequently the cost was equally small. Individuals in the career military service tended to remain on active duty for the maximum period of time so the size of the retired rolls was controlled in part by life expectancy. Coupled with this, the size of the active duty career military force was much smaller than that which is required today so the total number of potential retirees was smaller. Additionally the concept of youth and vigor has encouraged and/or forced early retirement with a larger number of retired military personnel who continue to receive retired pay for longer periods of time. Table 2.1 reflects the growth in size of the retired rolls between 1900 and 1960 by five year intervals.

Since the size of the military retired rolls increased beyond a quarter of a million persons in 1960, the cost of the program has become more critical. Table 2.2 provides figures regarding the size of the retired rolls and the costs for each year from 1960 to 1980.

The size of the retired rolls has quadrupled since 1960. In the same period of time annual costs have increased from approximately 700 million dollars to almost 12 billion dollars. These dollar figures are reflective of several factors such as active duty pay raises and consumer price index adjustments. Military retired pay is funded annually as a part of the Department of Defense budget from the general tax revenue. A multi-billion dollar payment program for individuals who

Table 2.1 Size of the Retired Rolls by Five-Year Intervals from 1900 to 1960

Year	Number
1900	3,029
1905	4,102
1910	5,405
1915	6,739
1920	10,035
1925	19,369
1930	32,838
1935	37,437
1940	48,374
1945	64,456
1950	132,828
1955	180,817
1960	255,089

Source: Actuarial Accountant of Office of Assistant Secretary of Defense for Manpower and Reserve Affairs

are no longer in uniform is not easily overlooked during the budgetary process. As a result considerable attention has been given during the past twenty years to annual monetary outlays to meet the retired payroll. Additionally, debate has arisen regarding the method of funding, which is now noncontributory, and the additive nature of the relationship of retired pay to social security benefits. The concept of youth and vigor has also been questioned seriously. All of the issues, however, appear to be aimed primarily at cost control and secondarily at the use of the retirement program as a personnel management tool.

Nondisability Retirement

Career military personnel become eligible for retirement after twenty years of active duty. There is no vesting so individuals who leave the uniformed services with less than twenty years have no equity in the retirement program. Upon retirement the individual begins an immediate annuity that lasts for the

Table 2.2 Size of Retired Rolls and Annual Budget, 1960–1980

Fiscal Year	Numbers	Fiscal Year budget ($ Millions)
1960	255,089	$ 0.693
1961	275,914	0.788
1962	331,436	0.896
1963	358,830	1.015
1964	410,853	1.211
1965	462,463	1.386
1966	508,566	1.592
1967	564,280	1.831
1968	624,496	2.093
1969	691,688	2.443
1970	750,144	2.853
1971	806,139	3.389
1972	867,190	3.889
1973	946,080	4.392
1974	1,017,271	5.137
1975	1,043,923	6.239
1976	1,096,184	7.300
1977	1,155,353	8.218
1978	1,192,055	9.173
1979	1,228,494	10.282
1980	1,264,525	11.919

life of the retiree. Retired pay is calculated on the basis of 2.5 percent of active duty basic pay multiplied by the number of years of military service, but not to exceed 75 percent of basic pay. For an individual who retires after twenty years, retired pay is 50 percent of basic pay and for the person who serves a full career of thirty years, retired pay is the maximum 75 percent of basic pay. Annuities, after retirement, automatically increase as the Consumer Price Index rises. Basic pay is only one component of regular military compensation; others are such things as housing allowance, food allowance, and special pay for hazardous duty or proficiency pay for highly skilled specializations. Retired pay for a typical enlisted person may be as little as about one-third of total active duty pay for a twenty-year retiree and about three-fifths for a thirty-year retiree (Hale, 1978).

Most career military personnel opt for the early retirement privilege. Approximately three-quarters of all enlisted retirees leave the service after twenty or twenty-one years. The typical twenty-year enlisted retiree is thirty-nine years of age at the time of retirement and will receive military retirement pay for thirty-three years before death. In 1978 dollars, the retiree will receive $190,000 in retired pay. About half of all officer retirees leave after twenty or twenty-one years service. Most officers leave involuntarily due to current tenure laws. The typical twenty-year retired officer is forty-three years of age at the time of retirement and will also receive pay for thirty-three years. In 1978 dollars retired pay will total $320,000 (Hale, 1978). At each age level the life expectancy for retired officers is longer than for enlisted personnel. Until about age sixty officers have a life expectancy of between three and one-half to four years longer than enlisted personnel. After age sixty this differential lowers to an average of two and one-half years and equals out at age eighty-five (Defense Manpower Data Center, 1981).

There has been considerable opposition and support for the early retirement feature. Most of the argument centers around five issues:

1. The need for a youthful and vigorous force to meet the demands of military duty.
2. The need to retain desired personnel.
3. The need to compensate individuals for the special institutional characteristics of military life (referred to as the X factor).
4. The need to provide a cushion to facilitate the transition to civilian life.
5. The need to avoid stagnation of rank in senior personnel and to enhance the promotional opportunity of junior personnel.

Persuasive arguments have been made on both sides of the early retirement issues. There seems to be some consensus that changes need to be made, but there is lack of agreement relative to amount of change and the aspects that should be changed.

Early retirement, however, poses special problems for the retiree that are created primarily because of the age at which retirement occurs. These aspects seem to get lost in the dialogue regarding the so-called liberality of the program. Retirement for individuals in most occupational groups occur at the "normal" retirement age of sixty-five. For these individuals living costs are usually reduced because they are beyond the age where major material acquisitions are being made and familial responsibilities are less than for younger parents. In contrast the recently retired military person has dependent, school-aged children or children in college. Because of frequent moves in the military service, they may be faced with purchasing a home at the time of retirement, thus increasing expenses even more. Both the retiree and family expect, or may demand, that they maintain an accustomed standard of living. In essence the retired military person may have the greatest need for financial resources at a time when income is being decreased because of retirement. Employment thus becomes a necessity for financial as well as for personal reasons. A forty-year-old retiree is a persona non grata in our culture. Usually the individual's self-esteem will not allow cessation from paid employment, but seeking employment at middle age often means being at a competitive disadvantage because of the years spent in the military service. Therefore, retirement takes an economic as well as a pychic toll. (The psychological impact of military retirement is treated in greater detail in Chapter 4.)

Retirement is a misnomer for the military retiree; a change of careers is probably a more accurate description. Most retirees do in fact seek full-time paid employment. There is some amount of controversy regarding how well the retiree fares economically in his quest to establish a second career. The University of Michigan Study published in 1960 reported that the typical retiree was at a decided disadvantage. The Michigan study found that for the typical retiree earnings from the second-career job and retired pay combined totaled less than the military person earned while on active duty or just equalled that amount (University of Michigan Study, 1961). A 1977 study by the Department of Defense found that the economic disadvantage continued to exist. The Department of Defense study compared first-job earnings of enlisted retirees with high school graduates and first-job earnings of officers with college graduates. Median educational level for enlisted personnel was high school graduate with 21 percent having more than a high school education. Educational level of the officers was some college with 21 percent having had graduate education. Age was held constant; forty to forty-nine for officers and their cohorts and thirty-five to forty-four for enlisted and their cohorts. Table 2.3 gives the results.

For officers there was an earnings differential of between 15 to 23 percent depending upon the year retired. For enlisted personnel the disparity ranged from 12 to 32 percent. With the enlisted retirees a striking trend appears; that is, the more recent the date of retirement, the greater the degree of disparity.

In 1981, R.V.L. Cooper of the Rand Corporation, under a contract with the Department of Defense, used the data from the 1977 DOD study and arrived at conclusions that were similar in some respects, but vastly different in others. Relative to reduced earnings Cooper found that officers earned 25 percent less than their nonretired, comparably aged and educated civilian peers while retired enlisted personnel earned about 20 percent less than their civilian peers. From this point on, however, Cooper differs with the Department of Defense study findings. He argues that it is by choice the military retiree earns less. The choices are related to decisions regarding the geographic selection of a retirement residence and an election to work less than full time. Because of their personal decision to retire in the South or West where there are "lower cost of living areas" and to accept lower paying jobs, their earnings would naturally be less. Cooper further states that even when retirees earn less, it is only for the first five years following their retirement (R.V.L. Cooper, 1981).

Table 2.3 First Job Earnings (Full Time Employed Mean Earnings in Dollars)

Year of retirement	Officer 1st job earnings	4 years college civilians	Difference between officers and 4 years college civilians	Percentage officer earnings of civilian counterparts
Age group 40–49 (officers)				
76	20,169[a]	23,701	3,532[a]	85.0[a]
74–75	17,889	21,804	3,915	81.6
72–73	14,745	19,284	4,539	76.4
70–71	13,184	16,781	3,597	78.5

Year of retirement	Enlisted 1st job earnings	Civilian high school graduates earnings	Difference between enlisted and high school graduates	Percentage enlisted earnings of civilian counterparts
Age group 35–44 (enlisted)				
76	10,112	14,905	4,793	68.0
74–75	10,720	13,817	3,097	77.5
72–73	9,901	12,358	2,457	80.1
70–71	9,468	10,746	1,278	88.1

[a]Based on sample size of 11

Source: Military Retiree Survey Report, 1978.

It appears to these writers that Cooper makes a far too simplistic argument. Multiple factors go into decisions regarding the selection of a retirement residence and the employment activity. Many retirees are influenced by family desires. For example, most retirees have school-age children and a major decision-making factor may be the children's insistence upon graduating from high school with their class. In a similar vein, the family may have established support systems in a particular community, often the locality of the last military assignment, and make a selection on this basis.

In terms of employment most retirees have not been able to secure sufficient financial resources to be very selective about job opportunities. Cooper himself writes that over 50 percent of retirees find employment in less than a month and 90 percent find employment in six months. In an earlier study McNeil found that the rapidity with which retirees found employment was indicative of their need to begin working immediately to maintain an accustomed standard of living (McNeil, 1964). Accepting a particular job may therefore be out of necessity and not out of a specific decision to take a low-paying job.

The fact that retirees earn less than their peers for five years following retirement is critical. These would be the readjustment and resettlement years when the need for high earnings is imperative. One can only speculate about the amount of time it takes one to catch up after having been at a competitive disadvantage for five years. It is quite possible the retiree would remain permanently at an economic disadvantage if the retired pay was not used to supplement income from post-retirement employment.

These studies indicate, however, that retired pay does in fact provide a cushion for the retiree in the transition to civilian life. Earnings from the civilian job and retired pay combined tends to decrease or remove the economic disadvantage and in some instances gives the retiree an economic edge in terms of gross income.

Disability Retired Pay

Disability retired pay refers to the annuity paid to members of the armed forces who are placed in retired status as a result of physical disability. Mental health disorders are included in this definition of physical disability. Nondisability retirement developed out of the history of disability pensions that were provided for military personnel who were injured in battle. Pensions are distinctly different from retirement pay. Retirement is reserved for those individuals who leave the military service voluntarily, involuntarily, or because of disability, but retain the right to benefits accorded to active duty personnel such as medical care, commissary, and base exchange privileges. The retired pay is funded through the military budget. Pensions, in contrast, are funded through the Veterans Administration and provide compensation for disability only. The veteran does not have privilege to military benefits. This discussion will focus primarily on the disability retired system and the veterans pension program will be mentioned only when necessary for clarity.

Disability retirement was embodied in the same piece of legislation that established the military retirement program in 1861. The initial disability retirement laws affected only officers; enlisted personnel were not included until 1941 (Third Quadrennial Review of Military Compensation, 1976).

Until 1941 disabled enlisted personnel were compensated through the veterans' pension system (*Hearings on . . . Gen. Earl E. Anderson,* 1975). Failure to include enlisted personnel who were disabled in the retirement program is reflective of the inequities in the program, which has attracted criticism over the years. Regular officers were treated more favorably than reserve officers and officers in one branch of the service were treated differently from officers in another branch (Third Quadrennial Review of Military Compensation, 1976; B. Cooper, 1970). Many of the inequities and inconsistencies were corrected in the Career Compensation Act of 1949 (63 U.S. Statutes, Section 802). Since before the turn of the century, officers who were disabled retired with 75 percent base pay and this procedure was continued for enlisted persons in the 1941 act. No attention was paid to the degree or severity of the disability or to its duration. The 1949 legislation established the system in operation today that addressed the degree of severity and the likelihood of permanency of the condition, and removed many of the inequities between categorics of officers and enlisted personnel.

Under the present system a military member who is unable to perform the duties of his office may be permanently retired for disability if two conditions are met: 1. if the disability is not the result of intentional misconduct or willful neglect and was not incurred during a period of unauthorized absence; and 2. the disability is rated at 30 percent or more or the member has at least twenty years of military service (Third Quadrennial Review of Military Compensation, 1976). The degree of disability is measured by using the Veteran's Administration schedule for rating disability. An individual retired for disability may select one of two ways to compute the amount of his compensation. Retired pay may be computed by multiplying the basic pay rate by the percentage of disability or by 2.5 percent of the number of years service. In either case the disability retired annuity may not exceed 75 percent of the member's active duty basic pay. Retired personnel may elect to receive whatever sum is greater. Another option available is that disability retirees may also elect to receive a Veteran's Administration pension in lieu of retired pay. Additionally the individual may receive a portion of his retired pay from the military service and the remainder from the Veteran's Administration. In these instances though, they retain all of the benefits and perquisites of a retired person. For lower-ranking personnel with limited military service time, it is usually more economically profitable for them to receive the veteran's pension.

All disabled individuals are not placed immediately on the permanent disability retired list. A member who would be qualified for permanent disability but for the fact that the permanency of his disability cannot be determined positively can be placed on the Temporary Disabled Retired List (TDRL). A member on TDRL has all of the retired pay entitlements as other retired persons, but there is a 50 percent floor on retired pay and the 75 percent ceiling remains. Individuals on the Temporary Disabled Retired List must receive a physical examination at least every eighteen months and some assessment made regarding the degree of impairment. A decision must be made within a period of five years whether or not the disability is permanent. If a periodic examination shows that the disability is permanent and it is rated as 30 percent or more, or if the member has at least twenty years service, the individual is placed on the permanent disability retired list. If the permanent disability designation is made and the degree of impairment is considered to be less than 30 percent, the member is removed from TDRL and paid disability severance pay. Severance pay is two months active duty basic pay for every year of military service up to a maximum of two years pay. Should it be determined the individual is physically able to perform military duty, the person may be voluntarily returned to active duty, but if this is refused the member is removed from the Temporary Disabled Retired List and retired pay is discontinued.

Disability retired pay is tax free. In contrast all other retired pay is subject to income taxation. Veteran's Administration pensions are also nontaxable.

Approximately 15 percent of the total retired population is comprised of disability retirees (Military Compensation Task Force, 1976). This percentage figure, however, has varied over the years from about 10 percent to almost 20 percent of the retired population. Periods during times of war and for a few years immediately afterward tend to be those instances when the number of disabled retirees is highest. Table 2.4 gives the average numbers of disabled retirees for the years 1972–1981 and the annual cost.

There have been no essential changes in the disability retired pay legislation since the Comprehensive Career Compensation Act of 1949. In 1956, however, when military service personnel began making contributions to the social security program

Table 2.4 Number of Disability Retirees, 1972–1981, and Cost

Year	Total personnel	Cost (in thousands of dollars
1972	153,929	631,127
1973	157,576	690,443
1974	159,384	754,761
1975	159,586	842,444
1976	159,532	919,532
1977	153,661	967,328
1978	152,780	1,025,203
1979	151,392	1,091,115
1980	149,768	1,196,473
1981	146,927	1,304,596

Source: The Budget of the U.S. Government, Fiscal Years 1974–1983.

they became eligible for social security benefits if they were permanently and totally disabled. This benefit is additive to disability retired pay.

Congress, though, has been quite vigilant in keeping informed of the number of career military persons who are placed on the disability retired list after they attain retirement eligibility on the basis of length of service. Disability retired pay, as indicated previously, is nontaxable, therefore it can be quite profitable to be found disabled at the time of retirement. There was evidence that officers were retired for disability at four times the rate for enlisted men. John J. Ford, professional staff member of House Armed Services Committee, reported prior to 1973 that 25 percent of all officers on the retired list were retired for disability, in contrast to 6 percent of enlisted personnel (*Hearings on . . . Gen. Earl E. Anderson,* 1975). Congressman Stratton (Democrat, New York), Chairman of the Subcommittee on Military Compensation of the House Armed Services Committee, expressed concern during the Vietnam War when Air Force General Lavelle was questioned "as to whether or not he had not conducted illegal bombing actions in Vietnam, he was found abruptly disabled after having served in a flight combat status, suddenly being disabled, I think, with a 70% disability. And as a result, a very major part of his $27,000 retired pay was tax free" (*Hearings on . . . Gen. Earl E. Anderson*, 1975). Disability retirement procedure was changed following the Lavelle incident, but surfaced again two years later when General Anderson, an unsuccessful candidate for the Marine Corps Commandant, was found 40 percent disabled when he applied for voluntary retirement after not being selected for the top position in the Marine Corps. Disability retirement for career military personnel has decreased considerably since 1975.

The Unfunded Liability

The military retirement system has always been a noncontributory program that is funded annually through congressional appropriations as part of the Department of Defense budget. When the nondisability retirement system was established during the Civil War the noncontributory practice that had been adopted for disability pensions was continued. Also continued was the procedure of paying for pension benefits out of the general tax revenue. Each year funds are appropriated by Congress for the Department of Defense and retirement costs are included in this budget. A pay-as-you-go system was therefore developed with the employer, the federal government, paying both the employee and employer share of retirement costs. On the surface, use of the term "noncontributory" appears accurate; however, military pay has been traditionally set lower than prevailing wages with the understanding that this reduced amount of pay was in lieu of a contributory retirement plan. There are advocates for contributory plans and their arguments may be summarized as follows:

1. Lower direct cost to the employer.
2. Possibility of a higher benefit level if an employee shares in the cost.
3. Greater understanding and appreciation of the retirement plan by the employee if he/she shares in the cost.

4. Belief that contributing a portion of the cost gives an employee a contractual right to the pension (University of Michigan Study, 1961).

The Michigan Study group evaluated each of these arguments. Relative to the issue of lower cost to the employer, they concluded that this is an illusory saving. Assuming the serviceman has contributed 6.5 percent of salary for a twenty-year period, the accumulated amount would be approximately 11 percent of the benefits eventually received. Additional costs would also be incurred. A contributory plan, when initially started, would require a raise in pay to avoid a reduction in take-home income. Individual accounts must be kept for each individual therefore increasing administration costs. Additionally only about 10 or 12 percent of the individuals who enter the military service remain until attaining retirement eligibility. Therefore, for almost 90 percent of military personnel a contributory plan would be simply a forced savings program. This argument regarding the illusory nature of savings does not include the value of interest that would be realized from investment of the fund in government bonds.

Benefit levels are not likely to be increased in face of a commonly held belief that pension benefits for the hazardous professions (military, policemen, and firemen) are already overly generous. The Michigan Study group found little cogency in the argument that military service personnel would have greater appreciation and understanding of their retirement system if it were contributory. Military personnel already have a good understanding and appreciation of their retirement program, in fact, more so than is the case with most other retirement systems.

Career military personnel already believe they have a contractual right to their pension. This right is established through congressional legislation mandating the development and implementation of a military retirement system. Attempts to alter the system have been contested in court, albeit not always successfully. One such case is the designation of military retired pay as community property in divorce cases (*McCarty* vs. *McCarty*, 1981).

The Michigan group concluded that Congress should not adopt a contributory retirement system for the military service (University of Michigan Study, 1961). Of the six or seven other major studies of military compensation, only two proposed a contributory system (Hale, 1978).

A more recent study evaluated the military retirement system and one of the issues focused upon was that of a contributory plan (Hale, 1978). The report acknowledges that a key reason for advocating a contributory retirement is to reduce cost. Such a system would reduce cost if a pay raise was not enacted to offset take-home pay lost when the contribution is deducted. A contribution with an offsetting pay raise would increase cost; however, a contributory system would make the military retirement program more consistent with the federal civil service program and other public sector plans. Hale also suggests a contribution would increase the plan's visibility and strengthen the contractual nature of it. Hale concluded, though, that there are major disadvantages to a contributory system. Without an offsetting pay raise all service personnel would have to absorb a pay reduction. Such a cut would exacerbate retention problems thus encouraging younger personnel to leave the military service and receive their refunds. Requiring a contribution would run counter to the practice in private industry where only about 20 percent of retirement plans are contributory. Moreover, military personnel already make an implicit contribution to their retirement program by accepting a depressed wage scale (Hale, 1978).

The noncontributory and pay-as-you-go features of the military retirement program have combined to develop an unfunded system. In recent years considerable attention has been paid to this "unfunded liability." The unfunded liability may be defined as the present value of prospective retired pay benefits over the sum of: 1. the amount in the pension fund, and 2. the present value of future contributions for normal cost (Church, 1979).

Several factors have brought attention to the unfunded liability. One obviously is the escalating cost of military retirement. Another factor arises out of the preoccupation over the unfunded liability of the federal social security system. Another grows out of the congressional effort to assure the stability of private pension plans. In 1974 the Employee Retirement Income Security Act (ERISA) was enacted as a reaction to the fact that many employees had lost pension rights because of bankruptcies, mergers, or ruthless employers (Church, 1979).

Movement, however, is in the direction of funded programs, not only in private plans, but public employees' plans also. Tilove (1976) has indicated that there was a massive movement away from pay-as-you-go plans about 1920 with a contrasting move toward actuarially computed reserve fund systems. Further, where unfunded public programs exist they are likely to have been inherited and authorities have not had the financial resources and the determination to change to a funded system. The military pay-as-you-go system was inherited, but it appears that there is currently some determination to change it to a funded plan. Tilove points out that simply moving to a funded plan does not completely solve the problem. It is possible to establish a fund that is only large enough to supplement benefit payments for a few years should cash flow problems develop.

At the other end of the continuum, it is possible to have a fully funded program with a reserve large enough to meet all future liability. Recommendations for a funded military retirement system seem to propose a plan that is inclined toward the fully funded end of the continuum. The fund would include sufficient resources to cover prior accrued liability in addition to future liability. Considering the number of active duty personnel in Fiscal Year 1981, 2,087,691, plus the number of retirees, 1,288,962, and the number of survivors' beneficiaries, 72,182 (Defense Manpower Data Center, 1981a), the size of the fund would be quite large. As of September 30, 1980, the entry-age, normal-cost unfunded liability was $431.1 billion (Defense Manpower Data Center, 1980).

One method of assessing the cost of retirement is looking at the projected unfunded liability. It is useful also, however, to examine retirement cost as a percentage of payroll.

A table prepared by actuaries at the Defense Manpower Data Center (shown in Table 2.5), projects this information over a seventy-five-year period, beginning in Fiscal Year 1980 and continuing to Fiscal Year 2055.

The ratio peaks at 65 percent of payroll in the year 2000 and then decreases to 54 percent in 2040 where it is expected to remain level. The actuaries indicate that under a funded entry-age, normal-cost method the ratio would be 46 percent. Additionally "a good argument for remaining unfunded could be made with only an 8 percent difference in ultimate budget outlays" (Defense Manpower Data Center, 1980).

To place the military retirement system on a funded basis necessitates amortizing the unfunded liability over a period of years. Table 2.6 indicates the additional monetary outlay, as a percentage of payroll, that would be required annually if the amortization is projected over a forty, fifty, or sixty-year period.

Although there appears to be a determination to change the current pay-as-you-go system to a funded program, there is a lack of clarity regarding the method of funding. Most of the major studies of military compensation have argued against contributions by the service person, but a contributory system has not been completely ruled out. If a contributory system were initiated, would the employee contribution be in addition to the social security deduction? A contribution in addition to the current 6.7 percent social security payroll tax (1982), assuming a 7 percent retirement deduction, would total almost 14 percent. On the other hand, if the contribution was included with the social security tax, again assuming 7 percent, the amount designated for the military retirement fund would be less than 1 percent.

A lack of clarity also exists regarding management of the fund. Undoubtedly the funds would be invested in government securities as is required with social security. Would the fund be managed by the Department of Defense or would the management function be the responsibility of some other existing or created federal agency?

Table 2.5 Total Past and Projected Basic Pay and Retired Appropriation Outlays[a] ($ in billions)

Fiscal Year	Total basic pay	Total retired appropriation outlays	Outlays/ payroll
1980[b]	$ 20.9	$ 11.9	0.5694
1981	23.5	13.9	0.5924
1982	26.8	15.6	0.5814
1983	29.3	17.2	0.5888
1984	31.6	18.8	0.5943
1985	33.7	20.2	0.5985
1986	35.8	21.6	0.6020
1987	37.9	22.9	0.6061
1988	40.0	24.4	0.6106
1989	42.2	26.0	0.6157
1990	44.5	27.6	0.6200
1991	47.0	29.4	0.6242
1992	49.6	31.2	0.6286
1993	52.3	33.1	0.6320
1994	55.2	35.0	0.6343
1995	58.3	37.1	0.6362
1996	61.5	39.2	0.6381
1997	64.8	41.5	0.6407
1998	68.3	43.9	0.6430
1999	72.0	46.4	0.6442
2000	75.9	48.9	0.6451
2005	98.8	63.1	0.6391
2010	128.9	80.1	0.6211
2015	168.5	100.7	0.5973
2020	220.4	127.1	0.5769
2025	288.0	161.9	0.5620
2030	376.4	207.9	0.5522
2035	491.9	268.6	0.5461
2040	642.9	348.8	0.5426
2045	840.3	454.5	0.5409
2050	1098.1	593.6	0.5405
2055	1435.4	775.9	0.5406

[a]Payroll projections include selected reserve and active duty basic pay, outlays include active duty and reserve retirements as well as survivor annuities
[b]Projected from this year on.

CPI Assumptions (Fiscal Year)

1981:	.095	1984:	.062
1982:	.087	1985:	.055
1983:	.073	1986 on:	.050

Salary Assumptions (Fiscal Year)

1982:	.143	1985:	.067
1983:	.092	1986:	.060
1984:	.078	1987 on:	.055

Source: Defense Manpower Data Center, 1980

Another issue is whether there even needs to be a retirement fund. Proponents of a pay-as-you-go system offer the following arguments (Tilove, 1976):

1. Pay-as-you-go involves the lowest immediate appropriation.
2. Increasing cost can be met more easily in the future, when dollars will be safer and the tax base larger.
3. Reserves are not necessary. Public authorities are bound to fulfill benefit commitments. Federal, state, and local governments are perpetual institutions that can tax to raise the money ultimately needed.
4. Reserves will only serve as a standing invitation to exact benefit increases that will absorb them.

Proponents of a funded system offer the following arguments (Tilove, 1976):

1. A funded system helps enforce responsibility in the following ways:
   a. allocated cost to the time the benefit is being accrued;
   b. increases the need for adequate cost accounting;
   c. minimizes the tendency to shift cost to a future generation.
2. Future generations may be unwilling to pay the cost of liability incurred by past generations.
3. A funded program reduces the cost because investment yields pay 25 to 50 percent of retirement benefits.
4. A funded system increases benefit security.

One writer has argued that "the uproar in recent years over increasing military retirement costs has been misguided because the costs will grow at less than 2 percent through the year 2000" (Church, 1979). As a consequence the size of the unfunded liability has been overemphasized (Church, 1979). Regardless of the arguments against a funded system, the move is in the direction of a funded plan. The Department of Defense is sponsoring legislation that would place the

Table 2.6 Military Retirement Appropriation Accrual Costs ($ in billions)

		Forty-year amortization as percent of payroll				
Year	Estimated[a] payroll	Normal cost	Payment on unfunded	Total accrual cost	Total estimated outlays	Added cost of accrual
1981	$ 23.5	$ 10.9	$ 11.86	$ 22.76	$ 13.9	$ 8.86
1982	26.8	12.4	12.51	24.91	15.6	9.31
1983	29.3	13.5	13.20	26.70	17.2	9.50
1984	31.6	14.6	13.93	28.53	18.8	9.73
1985	33.7	15.6	14.70	30.30	20.2	10.10
1986	35.8	16.5	15.51	32.01	21.6	10.41

		Fifty-year amortization as percent of payroll				
Year	Estimated[a] payroll	Normal cost	Payment on unfunded	Total accrual cost	Total estimated outlays	Added cost of accrual
1981	$ 23.5	$ 10.9	$ 9.70	$ 20.60	$ 13.9	$ 6.70
1982	26.8	12.4	10.23	22.63	15.6	7.03
1983	29.3	13.5	10.80	24.30	17.2	7.10
1984	31.6	14.6	11.39	25.99	18.8	7.19
1985	33.7	15.6	12.02	27.62	20.2	7.42
1986	35.8	16.5	12.68	29.18	21.6	7.58

Table 2.6, cont.

Year	Estimated[a] payroll	Sixty-year amortization as percent of payroll: Normal cost	Payment on unfunded	Total accrual cost	Total estimated outlays	Added cost of accrual
1981	$ 23.5	$ 10.9	$ 8.27	$ 19.17	$ 13.9	$ 5.27
1982	26.8	12.4	8.72	21.12	15.6	5.52
1983	29.3	13.5	9.20	22.70	17.2	5.50
1984	31.6	14.6	9.71	24.31	18.8	5.51
1985	33.7	15.6	10.25	25.85	20.2	5.65
1986	35.8	16.5	10.81	27.31	21.6	5.71

[a]Includes basic pay to active duty and selected reserves
Unfunded Liability 9/30/80 = $431.1 billion   Normal Cost[b] = .462
[b]Normal cost is computed as 46% of payroll and this remains constant throughout the period of amortization.

Source: Defense Manpower Data Center, 1980.

military retirement system on an entry-age, normal-cost funding method.

Integration with Social Security

Military personnel were not covered by social security with the act that was passed in 1935. Proposals were made during World War II to credit military service under the Social Security Act, but no coverage was authorized until 1946. This legislation provided for survivors of ex-servicemen who died within three years after they were discharged from the military service. The ex-serviceman must have served at least ninety days of active duty; however, the ninety-day minimum did not apply if he had been discharged for a service-connected disability. Survivor benefits were based upon an assumed wage of $160 per month. Funding for this survivor benefit was to be from the general tax revenue. This limited benefit was significant because it was gratuitous; it was prompted by concern for survivor benefits and was essentially a readjustment benefit for the service person. Much of the rationale upon which this beginning was made was that military service was a transient experience for most individuals who served on active duty, therefore, their time spent in the armed forces was an interruption of civilian employment. In August, 1950, legislation was enacted with a retroactive feature; all military service after September 15, 1941 and before July 25, 1947 was fully credited under Old Age and Survivors Insurance at a wage rate of $160 per month. As a result of this piece of legislation, survivors continued to be covered, but in addition the service person accrued retirement credits. Subsequent acts continued this coverage until 1957.

Survivor benefits again were the primary motivation for the 1957 law. Military personnel for the first time were brought into the social security system on a fully covered, participating basis. Gratuitous credits of $160 per month were no longer given. The service person contributed 50 percent of the social security tax, and the Department of Defense as employer contributed the other 50 percent. Old age insurance was to be additive at retirement age to any pension benefits to which the individual may have been entitled. Attention was so focused upon insuring survivor benefits that little if any thought was given to the impact of this legislation upon the military retirement system over the long term.

As the size of the retirement rolls have grown, more concern has been engendered about costs. An argument is made that the career service person gains entitlement to two pensions by virtue of one period of employment with the same employer. There is now widespread insistence that military retirement pension benefits be integrated with social security benefits when the retired military person begins receiving social security at age sixty-five, or sixty-two if an earlier retirement election is made. Each of the major studies of the military retirement system that has been made during the past ten or fifteen years has recommended some type of integration. At initial glance, integration appears straight forward and fair; however, closer inspection reveals some serious problems. These problems are related both to the nature of the social security retirement system and the methods of integration.

Social security was conceived as an omnibus program that sought to achieve two goals: 1. a welfare or income redistribution objective, and 2. a social insurance or earnings replacement objective. Although insurance terminology is used, it is primarily a tax and transfer system wherein current workers are taxed in order to provide benefits for those retired. The system maintains several trust funds that current workers replenish at the intake end and retired workers receive benefits at the disbursement end. This arrangement works reasonably well when there is a satisfactory ratio between replenishers and recipients. Second, the amount received should exceed, or at a minimum equal the amount disbursed. Supposedly there is an equitable relationship between the amount of money an individual deposits as a worker and the amount he receives as a retiree. This relationship is at best tenuous (Devine and Kuzmack, 1976).

INSURANCE OBJECTIVES.

The system is financed largely by a payroll tax levied upon employers and employees in equal percentages. As of January 1, 1982, the applicable tax was 6.7 percent of earnings on both employer and employee up to a wage ceiling of $32,400. Under present law both the tax and earnings ceiling are increased at designated intervals up to a maximum tax and celing of *7.65 percent* and *$42,600* respectively by 1990. Benefit levels are automatically increased on the basis of increases in the Consumer Price Index. According to the law, increases may not occur more frequently than annually. Congress, however, may alter this arrangement at any time (Devine and Kuzmack, 1976).

WELFARE OBJECTIVE.

Attempts to achieve welfare objectives are done in two ways. The first is the provision of benefits as an additive to the pension of the retired worker. If the retiree has a wife aged sixty-two or over, or if he has other dependents, they are entitled to benefits. The wage earner is the basic unit for taxation purposes, but the family is the basic unit for benefit purposes (Devine and Kuzmack, 1976).

A second attempt to achieve welfare objectives is through the relationship of prior earnings to benefits. In order to receive retirement benefits the wage earner must have been fully insured. To be fully insured the individual must have worked at least forty calendar quarters during which his covered earnings were at least $50 per quarter. Fifty dollars was the initial minimum earnings base per quarter, but as of January 1, 1982, this amount had increased to $340. Benefit levels are determined by summing the thirty-five years of highest earnings and dividing this total by 420 (the number of months in thirty-five years) to get the average monthly wage (AMW). Earnings in years other than the highest thirty-five are disregarded; if there are fewer than thirty-five years of covered earnings, a zero is entered in the numerator for the years of no covered earnings but the denominator remains 420.

After the above calculation, the primary insurance amount (PIA) is determined by reference to a table. Benefits are weighted so that lower-waged employees receive a higher proportion of their AMW than is the case for higher-waged employees. The weighting factor and the computational manner become very critical when integration of retired pay and social security benefits are considered for career military personnel (Devine and Kuzmack, 1976).

Integrated pension plans are those plans that take cognizance of social security benefits and treat them as a portion of the entire retirement package provided by the employer. Methods of integration may be implicit or explicit. Implicit integration plans simply set the scale of pension benefits lower than they would have been had there not been a social security pension benefit. Explicit integration means that a specified formula is developed to determine pension benefit levels that takes into account social security pension benefits. Explicit plans are of two general types: excess plans and offset plans. Excess plans have several variations, but a common characteristic is that the determination of benefits is based upon earnings above some specified level (e.g., the social security taxable wage ceiling). Offset plans subtract a certain percentage of the employee's social security benefit from his employer pension benefit. The most commonly used offset is 50 percent of the primary insurance amount (PIA), but it may go as high as 83.33 percent (Devine and Kuzmack, 1976).

The integration plan recommended by various groups that have studied the military retirement program has been the offset plan. Initiation of the offset plan had considerable support and in fact was included as a section of H.R. 7769 (The Uniform Services Retirement Modernization Act), which was introduced in Congress in June 1975. In preparation for congressional hearings, the Defense Manpower Commission was to prepare comments. Analysis of the offset provision, as recommended in the Retirement Modernization Act (RMA), revealed some unexpected and significant implications that had not previously been recognized. Previous proposals had recommended a 50 percent offset of that portion of the primary insurance amount (PIA) that was attributable to military service. The analysis

> found that an insoluble attribution problem exists under the current Social Security System; that is there is no method of unambiguously attributing a portion of an individual's Social Security benefit among employers when he has more than one employer. This problem arises both because of the structure of the formula relating benefits to average earnings and the method of calculating average earnings under the Social Security laws. . . . It was found that this is likely to deprive a retired member of a substantial portion of a Social Security benefit to which he would have been entitled based solely upon his civilian employment. To state it differently, the member will pay a substantial amount of Social Security taxes while in the military, yet under the offset provision his combined military retired pay and Social Security benefit will be lower than if he has never been covered by Social Security during military service. (Devine and Kuzmack, 1976)

Most retired military personnel have had more than one employer. Many armed forces personnel will have engaged in social security-covered employment prior to entering the military and a very large percentage will have "moonlighted" while on active duty. More than 75 percent of retired military personnel work full time after leaving the uniformed services. Depending upon the age at which they retire, the period of post-military civilian employment may exceed the total time spent in the military service. In most instances the employment will be in jobs that have social security coverage. The ambiguity and inequity of this situation is illustrated lucidly by Devine and Kuzmack (1976) through the use of varied case examples. Some of these case examples are reproduced below as "static" and "dynamic" cases. The first three are static cases.

A. Static Cases.

The three static cases all employ the following assumptions:

1. Money wages do not change. In all three cases military earnings are $6,000 every year; civilian earnings are $6,000

each year in the first case, $12,000 each year in the second, and $4,000 each year in the third.

2. The price level does not change.

3. The Social Security benefit table effective June 1, 1975 remains in effect throughout the period.

4. The maximum earnings subject to Social Security taxation remain at the 1975 level of $14,000 per year.

5. The 1975 Social Security tax rate of 5.85% (combined employer and employee rate of 11.7%) remains in effect.

Case 1

We shall discuss the first case to be analyzed in considerable detail for several reasons. It clearly indicates the nature of the attribution problem and it enables the reader to understand how the calculations were made. It also demonstrates the impact of the offset provision on the individual even under some very simple and unrealistic assumptions. We believe it will be clear that these assumptions understate the impact, i.e., that one may readily anticipate that the impact will be greater under the more realistic assumptions to be employed later. Subsequent cases will then be discussed more briefly.

In Case 1, we assume covered earnings of $6,000 per year during each of 20 years of military service, or total military covered earnings of $120,000. We also assume that the individual earns $6,000 per year in each of 20 years of civilian employment during his second career, and total civilian covered earnings are also $120,000. At age 65, the Social Security Administration would calculate his average monthly wage by selecting the 35 years during which covered earnings were highest, adding these, and dividing by 420 months. In this case, these earnings would total $210,000 (based upon 35 years at $6,000 per year). Dividing $210,000 by 420 resutls in an average monthly wage of $500; the current benefit table indicates a Social Security benefit of $323.40 for this AMW. Under the RMA offset procedure, he would have $120,000 of covered earnings during military employment; dividing this by 420 months results in an AMW of $285 and a PIA of $224.90 "attributable to military service." The offset would be 50% of the PIA, or $112.45.[1]

[1]The reader is reminded that this is a "static" case. The actual offset would not be based on the present benefit table, as in the example above, but on the benefit table when the member reaches age 65. The benefit table, and hence the offset, is likely to be substantially greater by then.

If we calculated the PIA "attributable to civilian employment" in the same manner, it would also be $224.90 based on his civilian employment alone; or, to put it another way, he would have received a PIA of $224.90 if he had never been covered by Social Security while in the military. The actual PIA which the individual receives from the Social Security Administration is $323.40 and military retired pay will be reduced by $112.45 at age 65, and the PIA minus the offset equals $210.95. However, he would be entitled to a PIA of $224.90 based upon his civilian employment alone. In this example, the sum of the individual's military retired pay and Social Security benefit at age 65 would be $13.95 per month *less* than it would have been had he not been covered by Social Security while in the military. Moreover, he would have paid over $7,000 in Social Security taxes during his military career, for which he would receive lower total retired pay than had he not paid these taxes.[2]

Case 2

We again assume that the member's covered earnings are $6,000 per year during each of 20 years of military service, but that they are $12,000 per year during each of 20 years of civilian covered employment. Total covered earnings are $120,000 in military employment and $240,000 in civilian employment. His AMW as calculated by the Social Security Administration would be $785 and his PIA would be $433.50. The AMW and PIA "attributable to military service" would be $285 and $244.90, respectively, and the offset would be $112.45, as in Case 1. The PIA less the offset ($433.50 minus $112.45) would be $321.05. However, he would have been entitled to a PIA of $356.90 based on his civilian employment alone. Therefore, the sum of his retired pay and Social Security benefit is $35.85 per month less than it would have been had he not been covered by Social Security while in the military, and he would have paid over $7,000 in Social Security taxes during military employment.

[2]Throughout our static analysis we assume the present Social Security tax rate of 5.85% each for employer and employee. Actually, the rate is scheduled to increase under current law to 6.05% in 1978, 6.3% in 1981, and 6.4% in 1986.

Case 3

In this case we again assume earnings of $6,000 during each of 20 years of military employment and we assume covered earnings of $4,000 during each of 20 years of civilian employment. Total covered earnings are $120,000 in military employment and $80,000 in civilian employment. Both annual and total covered earnings in civilian employment are two-thirds those in military employment. The actual PIA would be $292.40 and the offset is $112.45; the PIA less the offset is $179.95, or $0.95 less than the PIA of $180.90 to which he would have been entitled based upon his civilian employment alone.

In addition to demonstrating the attribution problem, a general principle emerges from consideration of these three static cases; namely, the higher the proportion of covered earnings in civilian employment to covered earnings in military employment, the more adverse the impact of the offset on the member.

B. Dynamic Cases

It was necessary to make numerous assumptions in analyzing the dynamic cases. We believe that we have generally made "conservative" assumptions, i.e., assumptions which minimize the adverse impact of the offset provision of the RMA.

For the period 1957–1975, military covered earnings were based on typical promotion profiles, the prevailing pay tables, and a gratuitous Social Security wage credit of $1,200 per year when applicable. Prevailing Social Security tax rates and ceilings were also used. Historical earnings were used to develop more realistic earnings profiles than were used in the static case. However, it is assumed that the RMA was in effect throughout the entire period.

For future periods, we assumed a 3% annual increase in the Consumer Price Index. The benefit table was increased consistent with this assumption and with the provisions of law governing the method and timing of such increases. Military base pay, civilian earnings, and average taxable wages reported to the Social Security Administration were assumed to increase at a rate of 5% per year. Projected increases in the ceiling on covered earnings and maximum average monthly wages for benefit determination were made consistent with this assumption and the applicable provisions of law, beginning in 1977. (The ceiling was assumed to be $15,300 for 1976.) We assumed no legislated changes in the benefit tables or ceilings; i.e., all changes were in accordance with the automatic provisions of the Social Security laws. The Social Security tax rate was assumed to remain at 5.85%.

Case 4

An officer enters the military on January 1, 1957 and retires on December 31, 1976 as an O-5 with 20 years of service. His covered earnings have been above the then current ceilings for Social Security taxation since early in his career. His base pay upon retirement is $22,559 per year, well above the 1976 ceiling of $15,300. We assume a second career of 20 years in covered employment and retirement upon reaching age 62. Covered earnings during these years are the same as the Social Security ceiling, which increases at the rate of approximately 5% per year.

The pertinent summary data are:

	Military	Civilian	Lifetime
Years covered	20	20	40
Covered earnings	$148,249.56	$536,400.00	$684,649.56
Average monthly wages	$352.98	$1,277.14	$1,577.14
Primary insurance amount	$524.10	$1,105.20	$1,218.50

Offset = $262.05
PIA minus offset = $956.45
Monthly decrease = $148.75

It should be noted that the PIA's shown are those which will be in effect when the officer is 65 in the year 2000, based on the assumed increase in the benefit table. The average monthly wage attributable to military service is $352.98. However, the PIA associated with the wage will be $524.10 in the year 2000; the offset will be 50% of this PIA, or $262.05. The PIA of $1,218.50 minus the offset equals $956.45. He would have been entitled to a PIA of $1,105.20 based on his civilian employment alone. Therefore, the sum of the member's retired pay and Social Security benefit will be $148.75 per month less than the sum of retired pay plus the Social Security benefit to which he would have been entitled solely on the basis of his civilian employment. During his military career, he would have paid $6,815 in Social Security taxes.

The member's retired pay in the year 2000 will be approximately $2,300 per month under the present method of adjusting retired pay, and the offset of $262 will be about 11% of retired pay. The offset will be 14% of his final year's base pay, which is substantially higher than the 4% estimated by DOD. However, the DOD estimates were made under different assumptions which are both unrealistic and inconsistent with the automatic provisions of the Social Security Act Amendments of 1972 for adjusting benefits and ceilings.

If the offset at age 65 were based on the PIA in effect when he retired on December 31, 1976, as is required of private employers under the Employee Retirement Income Security Act of 1974 (ERISA), then it would be $132.80 instead of $262.05. Nevertheless, the decrease in the individual's total retired pay because of offsetting would be $19.50 per month. This indicates that the same problem can arise in the private sector when an individual has multiple employers.

Case 5

An officer enters the military on January 1, 1957 and retires on December 31, 1986 as an O-6 with 30 years of service. His base pay is calculated from actual pay tables until October 1, 1976, and projected to increases at 5% per year thereafter. We assume a second career of 10 years in covered employment and retirement upon reaching age 62. Covered earnings during these years are the same as the Social Security ceiling.

The pertinent summary data are:

	Military	Civilian	Lifetime
Years covered	30	10	40
Covered earnings	$352,549.56	$332,100.00	$684,649.56
Average monthly wage	$839.40	$790.71	$1,577.14
Primary insurance amount	$907.90	$883.50	$1,218.50

Offset = $453.95
PIA minus offset = $764.55
Monthly decrease = $118.95

His PIA of $1,218.50 less the offset of $453.95 equals $764.55. He would have been entitled to a PIA of $883.50 based solely upon his civilian employment. The sum of his retired pay and Social Security benefit is $118.95 per month less than it would have been if he were not covered by Social Security in the military. This is not as large as the decrease of $148.75 per month in Case 4 because a smaller proportion of the O-6's lifetime covered earnings were in civilian employment.

However, he would have paid $18,766 in Social Security taxes during his military career compared with $6,815 for the O-5 who retired after 20 years, even though both had the same earnings for the first 20 years. The additional taxes resulting from the last 10 years of service ($11,951) are disproportionately large because of increases in the maximum earnings subject to Social Security taxation.

If the offset at age 65 were to be based on the PIA in effect when he retired at age 52, as required of private employers under ERISA, then it would be $309.10 instead of $453.95. In this case, the sum of his retired pay and Social Security would be $25.90 per month higher than if he had not been covered by Social Security while in the military, a small increment in view of the additional taxes paid.

Case 6

An enlisted man enters the military on January 1, 1957 and retires on December 31, 1976 as an E-7 with 20 years of service. This case approximates the experience of a majority of military retirees. During the period 1960–1975 about 78% of military retirees were enlisted personnel, and the average years of service and pay grade upon retirement for these personnel is 21 years and E-7, respectively. We assume a second career of 24 years in covered employment and retirement upon reaching age 62. His second career earnings are assumed to begin at $9,500 and increase at a rate of 5% per year thereafter. His covered earnings are below the maximum for Social Security taxation during all years of his military and civilian employment.

The pertinent summary data are:

	Military	Civilian	Lifetime
Years covered	20	24	44
Covered earnings	$121,196.14	$422,769.00	$543,965.14
Average monthly wage	$288.56	$1,006.59	$1,222.82
Primary insurance amount	$520.10	$1,114.50	$1,218.80

Offset = $260.05
PIA minus offset = $958.75
Monthly decrease = $155.75

His PIA of $1,218.80 minus the offset of $260.05 equals $958.75. He would have been entitled to a PIA of $1,114.50 based solely upon his civilian employment. The sum of his retired pay and Social Security is $155.75 per month less than it would be if he were not covered by Social Security while in the military. If the offset were restricted to 50% of the PIA in effect at the time he retired (as would be required under ERISA), then this sum would be $12.80 per month less than if the military employment were not covered by Social Security.

Case 7

Thus far we have analyzed the effect of the offset on the total of the member's retired pay and PIA, and not necessarily on the total benefit received from Social Security. However, if the member is married, his wife will become entitled to a wife's benefit equal to 50% of his PIA when she reaches 65. The offset is applied only to the PIA, as is also true in the private sector under Internal Revenue Service rules.

We analyze the effect of the offset on the sum of retired pay, the PIA, and the wife's benefit, using the data from Case 6. The member receives a PIA from the Social Security Administration of $1,218.80; when his wife reaches age 65, she will be entitled to a benefit of $609.40, for a total of $1,828.20. The total benefit minus the offset of $260.05 equals $1,568.15. Based upon civilian employment alone, the member would be entitled to a PIA of $1,114.50; the wife's benefit would be $557.15 and the total would be $1,671.75. The sum of retired pay, the PIA, and the wife's benefit, therefore, would be $103.60 per month less (compared with $155.75 less in Case 6) than if the member were not covered by Social Security while in the military.

The adverse impact of the offset is therefore ameliorated, although still substantial. This amelioration depends upon three assumptions: (1) that the member has a wife; (2) that she is at least 65; and (3) that she is not entitled to a higher benefit based upon her own labor force participation. To the extent that wives of enlisted men are more likely to be entitled to a benefit in their own right, the offset provision will be a greater disadvantage to enlisted members than officers (see Table 2.7).

Analysis of the offset provision as proposed in the Retirement Modernization Act stopped legislative action to integrate retired pay with social security. The concept of integration, however, persisted and was recommended again by the President's Commission on Military Compensation in their 1978 report. The commission recommended an offset formula. At age sixty-five, or sixty-two if social security is elected early, military retired pay would be reduced by 1/25 percent of the initial social security primary insurance amount (PIA) for each

Table 2.7 Summary of Results of Cases Analyzed

Case Number[a]	Years of covered employment		Covered earnings		Monthly decrease[b]
	Military	Civilian	Military	Civilian	
1	20	20	$120,000	$120,000	$ 13.95
2	20	20	120,000	240,000	35.85
3	20	20	120,000	80,000	0.95
4	20	20	148,250	536,400	148.75
5	30	10	352,550	332,100	118.95
6	20	24	121,196	422,769	155.75
7[c]	20	24	121,196	422,769	103.60

[a]Static assumptions used for Cases 1–3 and dynamic assumptions for Cases 5–7.
[b]Amount by which the sum of military retired pay and PIA to which member would be entitled based solely upon civilian employment exceeds the sum of military retired pay and PIA under Social Security offset, except for Case 7 (See footnote 3.).
[c]Same earnings pattern as Case 6, but the sum of PIA plus 50 percent wife's benefit is used instead of PIA.

Source: Devine and Kuzmack, 1976.

Table 2.8 Effect of Social Security Offset on Retired Pay at Age 65 for Person Leaving Active Duty in 1978

Grade	Years of service	Percentage reduction in military retired pay at age 65 due to social security offset[a]
O-5	20	17.4
E-7	20	34.3
O-5	25	13.1
E-8	25	26.6
O-6	30	11.2
E-8	30	20.0

[a]Social security benefits were calculated using the provision of the 1977 Social Security Act amendments, assuming an individual will collect social security benefits in the future at age 65. Military covered earnings were based on average enlisted and officer career paths; civilian covered earnings were based on the median income of high school graduates for enlisted persons and the median income of college graduates for officers assuming a 1.5 percent annual real wage growth.
Source: Report of President's Commission on Military Compensation, 1978.

year served in the uniformed services. Approximately two-thirds of the corporate pension plans that use a graduated offset procedure use one similar to this one (Bankers Trust Company, 1975). In no case would the reduction exceed 50 percent of an individual's military retirement paycheck. The commission formula took specific cognizance of the fact that the typical retiree has had two or more employers during a work career. Additionally the formula recognizes that the service member has paid half of the social security contribution. The provision is designed to produce a 50 percent offset for a person who has a forty-year work career. Individuals who work less than forty years would have proportionately smaller offsets. Because of the social weighting of social security benefits, enlisted personnel would have a larger percentage

Table 2.9 Percentage of After-Tax Active Duty Income Replaced by After-Tax, Military Retired Pay and Social Security at Age 65: Commission Plan[a]

Rank	Years of service	Percent
E-7	20	78.5
O-5	20	65.8
E-7	22	77.5
O-5	22	68.6
E-8	25	78.0
O-6	25	73.4
E-8	30	85.6
O-6	30	81.7

Source: Report of President's Commission on Military Compensation, 1978

offset than officers (*Report of the President's Commission on Military Compensation*, 1978). A sampling of these percentage differences is reflected in Table 2.8.

Although Table 2.8 reflects a disproportionately larger offset for enlisted personnel when military retired pay and the social security annuity are combined, officers realize a smaller percentage of their after-tax active duty pay (see Table 2.9).

Which ever integration method is used, the retired service person will realize a smaller annuity once social security retirement benefits are received. As reflected by the preceding discussion these reductions could be substantial. Either method would, in the long run, help reduce the cost of military retirement. Cost reduction is not the only reason offered for integration, however, it does appear to be a strong motivator. Problems such as those previously detailed have delayed action regarding integration and the remaining factors that must be considered in any plan to modify the military retirement program. Integration should not be pursued independently but as part of a complete overhaul or modification. When and if integration is achieved there is no way of doing so without creating some degree of inequity. The integration plan selected hopefully will minimize the amount of inequity. Kuzmack has concluded that there is no analytical solution to the integration of social security with other pensions. The solution must be an essentially political one, and compromises will have to be made (Kuzmack, 1978).

This treatise focuses upon the retired military person; however, it is obvious that the same inequities would occur in the civilian labor market for an individual who has had more than one employer during a lifetime work career.

Survivor Benefits

Before the passage of the Uniformed Services Contingency Option Act of 1953, there were no provisions to allow a retired serviceman to leave a portion of his retirement annuity upon his death to a surviving spouse or dependent children. Retirement pay was considered to be the sole property of the retired serviceman and was discontinued at the time of his death. As a result many surviving widows discovered to their dismay that they were in severe financial straits. Widespread recognition of the destitution of these surviving widows led to the passage of the Contingenty Option Act in 1953 where a retired military member could elect to receive reduced retirement pay during his lifetime so as to entitle his survivors to an annuity after death. Although there was great need for the program, very few military persons subscribed to it because of the high cost and restrictive features, which were related to the fact that the program had to be actuarially neutral. The law specifically provided that the survivorship annuity program had to be completely self-financing by the contributions of participating members. Administration costs, however, were paid by the federal government (Third Quadrennial Review of Military Compensation, 1976). Among the specific unattractive features were:

1. It was expensive; for example the cost per dollar of coverage for a forty-five year old nondisability retiree with a forty year old wife was 22.8 cents per dollar of coverage.
2. Contributions were subject to taxation, so taxes were paid on money never received.
3. Election had to be made prior to the eighteenth year of active duty, so a decision had to be made for a program that perhaps would not take effect for twelve years.
4. If the beneficiary died before the retiree, annuity payments continued (Third Quadrennial Review of Military Compensation, 1976).
5. Revocation of participation in the plan was practically impossible.

Because of these unattractive features, participation in the plan never exceeded 15 percent (Third Quadrennial Review of Military Compensation, 1976). A number of changes were made over the next several years in order to liberalize the program and improve its image; however, the self-supporting mandate remained intact. In 1961 the name was changed from Contingency Option to the Retired Serviceman's Family Protection Plan (RSFPP). Flexibility was introduced by permitting such things as elections to be made after the eighteenth year of service, but the military member must remain on active duty for three years for it to be effective, and authorizing revocation of coverage because of "extreme financial hardship," but approval of the Branch of Service Secretary was required. The actuarial neutrality of the RSFPP was retained and the cost was increased even more. Now the forty-five year old retiree with a wife five years younger had to pay 25.3 cents per dollar of coverage. Participation remained low. The year 1966 brought about other changes. The amount by which retired pay was reduced because of participation in RSFPP was declared exempt from income taxation. Participation again remained at a totally unsatisfactory low level.

Attempts were therefore made to reduce the degree of restrictiveness additionally in a 1968 change in the law. Elections to participate in RSFPP could be made after the nineteenth year of active duty and the election could become effective immediately. The act reduced from three to two years the period of subsequent active duty required to make a post-nineteen-year election, change, or revocation effective. Approval of the service secretary was no longer required for revocation or reduction of annuity; however, a six-month delay was imposed. Elections could be for annuities of any amount between 55 and 12.5 percent in contrast to the previous one-half, one-fourth, or one-eighth of retired pay.

These liberalizing features did increase significantly the flexibility of RSFPP, but since it remained self-supporting, costs soared. The hypothetical forty-five year old husband with a forty year old wife must now pay 42.9 cents per dollar of coverage (Third Quadrennial Review of Military Compensation, 1976). None of these peripheral changes raised the participation rate above approximately 15 percent. Therefore 85 percent of the spouses of retired armed forces personnel had no entitlement in the retirement annuity of the service person. There was continuing and increased pressure from affected survivors and national organizations for fundamental changes in the Retired Serviceman's Family Protection Plan. Some of the organizations pressing for change were the Air Force Sergeants Association, the Retired Officers Association, the National Association for the Uniformed Services, the Disabled Officers Association, the American Legion, and the Military Wives Association. Several Congressmen were sympathetic and supportive of the dire need for change.

As a result of this concern, Congress in 1970 began a "comprehensive inquiry into the question of the adequacy of existing survivor benefit programs for dependents of the members of the Armed Forces, active & retired" (Hearings, *Report of the Special Subcommittee on Survivor Benefits,* 1970). During the latter years of this imbroglio, increased attention was given to the idea of attaining some comparability of compensation and benefits between the federal civil service system and the military service. During the hearings, several individuals testified about the disparity between the two programs. A major difference in the two programs is that the government shares in the cost of the civil service plan whereas the military survivor program was self-supporting. The participation rate in the civil service plan was 90 percent in contrast to the 15 percent participation rate in RSFPP (*Hearings, Report of the Special Subcommittee on Survivor Benefits,* 1970). Table 2.10 reflects the cost differences using 1970 salary scales.

The retired military person pays more than twice as much and at some points almost quadruple the amount of premium for a smaller annuity. It appeared the time had arrived for fundamental changes in the method of financing survivor benefit annuities for dependents of retired military personnel. Congressional hearings began on July 7, 1970 (Hearings, *Report of the Special Subcommittee on Survivor Benefits,* 1970) that eventuated in the enactment of the Survivor Benefit Program, which was signed into law on September 21, 1972.

Four primary purposes were explicated in the philosophical basis for the proposed bill. They were:

1. Provide a fair level of income replacement for survivors.
2. Call for some cost sharing at a reasonable level by the retiree that would meet the government's obligation to survivors and still be acceptable in terms of financial demands upon the government.
3. A plan that could be generally applicable to all military retirees.
4. A plan that could be easily understood by the retirees and their dependents.

The bill therefore proposed governmental participation in sharing the cost of the program. Emphasis was placed upon making the program reasonably comparable to the civil service survivor annuity plan. There was controversy over whether benefits should be integrated with social security or should be an add-on similar to civil service and the military retirement program. The supporters of integration and an offset provision

Table 2.10 Cost Comparison of Civil Service and RSFPP Survivor Programs

Grade	Years of service	Monthly base pay	Monthly retired pay	Age at retirement	Amount of RSFPP annuity (50 percent)	Cost[a]	Civil service annuity (55 percent)	Cost[b]
E-5	20	$ 451.80	$ 225.90	40	$112.95	$ 20.18	$124.25	$ 5.65
E-6	21	532.50	279.56	41	139.78	26.31	153.76	6.99
E-7	22	645.60	355.08	42	177.54	35.19	195.29	13.01
E-7	30	726.30	544.73	50	272.37	80.49	299.60	31.97
O2E[c]	24	847.50	508.50	47	254.25	64.91	279.68	28.35
O3E[c]	26	1,001.10	650.72	47	325.36	83.06	357.90	42.57
O-4	28	1,140.30	798.21	47	399.11	101.89	439.02	57.32
O-6	30	1,671.30	1,253.48	50	626.74	185.20	689.41	102.85
O-8	30	2,188.20	1,641.15	52	820.58	266.85	902.63	141.62

[a]Cost of RSFPP premium based on man's age, spouse 5 years younger with children.
[b]Cost of beneficiary's annuity under civil service retirement system.
[c]4 years' prior enlisted service

Source: Hearings, *Report of The Special Subcommittee on Survivor Benefits of the Committee on Armed Services,* 1970 prevailed. It was hoped that participation would reach the 85 percent level.

Major provisions of the 1972 Survivor Bill (SBP) are:

1. Members of the armed forces with eligible dependents who retired after enactment of the bill are automatically enrolled at the maximum (55 percent) level unless the individual specifically declines in writing.
2. If less than maximum coverage is desired, any base amount between $300 and the entire retired pay of the member may be selected.
3. Cost for spousal coverage is 2.5 percent of the first $300 of the base amount plus 10 percent of the remainder of the base amount.
4. Cost for children coverage is determined actuarially.
5. Premium and annuity amounts are adjusted in accordance with the Consumer Price Index (CPI).
6. A member without dependents may buy an annuity for someone with an insurable interest in him/her.
7. The SBP is integrated with social security and requires a reduction in payments when the survivor is eligible for social security. The annuity is reduced by that portion of the member's social security benefit that is attributable to active military service.
8. A gratuitous guaranteed minimum income is provided for "low income widows."
9. The survivor of a member who dies while in active duty after attaining retirement eligibility is eligible for an annuity at the same level as if the member had contributed to the program (Third Quadrennial Review of Military Compensation, 1976).

These changes did in fact increase participation. By September 30, 1979, there was a 51 percent participation rate (Hearings, *Benefits for Survivors of Retired Military Personnel*, 1980). In Fiscal Year 1981 the participation rate was 50 percent (Defense Manpower Data Center, 1981). Decreased cost to the member and increased flexibility in the plan no doubt

Table 2.11 Cost Comparison: Military vs Civil Service

Cost of living increases	Survivor annuity	Monthly Cost: Military	Monthly Cost: Civil service
—	$165.00	$ 7.50	$ 7.50
Jul 73 - 6.1%	175.00	9.33	7.96
Jan 74 - 5.5%	184.70	11.80	8.40
Jul 74 - 6.3%	196.52	13.20	8.93
Jan 75 - 7.3%	210.67	15.80	8.58
Aug 75 - 5.1%	221.41	17.76	10.06
Mar 76 - 5.4%	233.41	19.93	10.60
Mar 77 - 4.8%	244.57	21.97	11.11
Sep 77 - 4.3%	255.08	23.88	11.59
Mar 78 - 2.4%	261.21	24.99	11.87
Sep 78 - 4.9%	274.00	27.32	12.45
Mar 79 - 3.9%	284.70	29.26	12.95
Sep 79 - 6.9%	304.34	32.83	13.85
Mar 80 - 6.0%	322.60	36.15	14.68
Total annuity cost (June 1973 - June 1980)		$1,789.29	925.56
Additional cost to military retiree for identical coverage:		$ 863.73	

Assumption: Both retirees left Federal Service on June 1, 1973 and elected identical survivor annuity coverage.

Source: Hearings, *Benefits for Survivors of Retired Military Personnel,* 1980

contributed to this change, but probably significant was the fact that election of the annuity was automatic unless specifically refused. Although there was cost-sharing by the government and the member, the premium for the survivor annuity was more expensive for the military retireee than for the civil service retiree, as reflected in Table 2.11.

In spite of improvements in the Survivor Benefit Plan (SBP), some unattractive features remained. Most prominent among the unpopular aspects was the social security offset. At age sixty-two, if the survivor was drawing the annuity, it was offset by 100 percent of the social security benefit attributable to active duty military service. In some instances this could erase the entire SBP annuity or at least a large percentage of the benefit (Retirement Supplement, *Army Times,* July 12, 1982).

In the examples used in Table 2.12, the social security offset represented a considerable reduction in the amount of the annuity received by the survivor. The survivor of an E-7, for example, who retired in 1965 would suffer a $210.00 monthly offset, thereby receiving an annuity of only $114.00.

The next most unattractive feature was the method used to recompute the retiree's contribution to the SBP program each time there was a Consumer Price Index adjustment. Due to a defect in the recomputation formula, the contribution of the member increased at a faster rate than the real percentage of the survivor annuity (Retirement Supplement, *Army Times,* July 12, 1982). The other most persistent irritant dealt with the nonrevocation clauses. Deductions from retired pay continued if the beneficiary died, if there was a divorce, or if the member became disabled from a service-connected injury or disease and no longer needed SBP because the spouse was covered under the Veteran's Administration Dependency and Indemnity Compensation (DIC). (The latter is a noncontributory program.) Should the survivor receive DIC payments, the SBP annuity would be offset by that amount even though the offset could totally reduce the SBP annuity (Retirement Supplement, *Army Times,* July 12, 1982). These dissatisfactions and inequities led to further review of the Survivor Benefit Plan.

Table 2.12 Examples of Survivor Benefits

Year of retirement	Paygrade at retirement	Years of service at retirement	Social security offset	No offset	1972 law offset
1965	E-7	20	$210.00	$ 324.00	$ 114.00
	E-8	25	218.00	493.00	275.00
	E-9	30	203.00	736.00	533.00
	O-5	20	216.00	695.00	479.00
	O-5	25	231.00	1,046.00	815.00
	O-6	30	223.00	1,362.00	1,139.00
1980	E-7	20	315.00	307.00	—0—
	E-8	25	365.00	466.00	101.00
	E-9	30	400.00	695.00	295.00
	O-5	20	398.00	656.00	258.00
	O-5	25	424.00	988.00	564.00
	O-6	30	423.00	1,286.00	863.00

Note: Benefits in constant 1980 dollars, 100 percent coverage

Source: Hearings, *Benefits for Survivors of Retired Military Personnel,* 1980

Additional improvements have been made in the program, the most recent being in 1981. Primarily attention was given to removing inequities. For example, previously there was a social security offset for a widow with one child, but none if there were two or more children. There is no longer the offset regarding children. Previously there was also an offset when social security earnings were based upon the survivor's own earnings record. Problems of this sort in the SBP were corrected; however, the entire issue of the social security offset remains. A partial resolution, though, was reached. Congressman Wilson (Democrat, California) member of the House Armed Services Committee argued for a 50 percent offset rather than the 100 percent offset (Hearings, *Benefits for Survivors of Retired Military Personnel,* 1980). The eventual compromise was that "Social Security benefits to a surviving spouse may reduce the SBP benefit no more than 40%." Thus a beneficiary is assured of at least 60 percent of the annuity that the deceased spouse purchased. Comparisons of the annuity amounts utilizing the different formulas are shown in Table 2.13. The 50 percent social security offset would be more favorable for the beneficiary than the 40 percent cap in each instance, except for the lowest annuity payment.

Arguments supporting a social security offset generally center around the fact that the government, as employer, pays for one-half of the social security premium. If the benefit is not offset the beneficiary would receive two annuities from the same contribution. A counterargument is that if there must be an offset it should be restricted to 50 percent rather than the 100 percent formula since the service person pays the other 50 percent of the premium. When the civil service comparability issue is raised it is pointed out that the federal civil servants are not covered by social security. Approximately 80 percent of federal civil servants do qualify for social security benefits by virtue of moonlighting or working in private employment at other times in their working lifetimes. As a result many, therefore, receive very significant windfalls, (Hearings, *Benefits for Survivors of Retired Military Personnel,* 1980).

Table 2.13 Cost Projections For SBP Example Survivor Benefit Annuities

				Amount survivor receives								
				Full Coverage[a]			Typical Coverage[b]			Minimum coverage		
Year of retirement	Rank	Years of service	Social security offset[c]	No offset	50 percent offset	40 percent max. reduction	No offset	50 percent offset	40 percent max. reduction	No offset	50 percent offset	40 percent max. reduction
1980	E-7	20	$287	$ 300	$ 157	$180	$ 240	$ 97	$144	$165	$22	$99
	E-9	30	357	672	514	403	470	292	282	165	0	99
	O-5	20	345	654	482	392	491	319	294	165	0	99
	O-6	30	383	1,244	1,052	861	995	803	612	165	0	99
1990	E-7	20	278	325	186	195	260	121	156	89	0	53
	E-9	30	402	727	526	436	509	308	305	89	0	53
	O-5	20	413	708	502	425	531	325	319	89	0	53
	O-6	30	513	1,346	1,090	808	1,077	821	646	89	0	53
2000	E-7	20	276	341	203	205	273	135	164	55	0	33
	E-9	30	397	763	564	458	534	335	320	55	0	33
	O-5	20	408	742	538	445	557	353	334	55	0	33
	O-6	30	560	1,412	1,132	852	1,130	850	678	55	0	33

[a]Look back and save-pay provisions not included.
[b]Percent covered varies with rank and years of service.
[c]Wage growth included to retirees age 62 then brought back to 1980 dollars by inflation. Amount shown assumes beneficiary's offset occurs at age 62 and is therefore .829 of the primary insurance amount attributable to military service.

Note: Constant 1980 dollars, post-1985 inflation/wage growth = 5–5.5 percent

Source: Hearings, *Benefits for Survivors of Retired Military Personnel,* 1980

In view of the fact that currently only one-half of retirees subscribe to SBP, there is reason to believe that some of the features are still considered to be quite undesirable. Officers participate at a rate approximately twice that of enlisted personnel.

Restrictive Legislation

Two pieces of legislation enacted in the 1890s had a profound impact upon the post-retirement employment of military personnel, especially retired regular officers. They were the Dual Office Act (later changed to Dual Compensation) of 1894 and the Conflict of Interest Statute of 1896. The Dual Compensation Act has received the most national attention over the past fifteen to twenty years.

The Dual Office Act of 1894 provided that no person, including retired regular military officers, could hold two federal offices if the annual salary of either was $2,500 or more. Retired regular officers were considered to hold a federal office as a result of their having been tendered a regular commission while on active duty. When the legislation was passed, congressmen earned $5,000 per year and the highest level federal civil service employees earned $2,500. The effect of the legislation was that no federal employee could earn as much or more than a member of Congress. Relatively few military retirees were affected in 1894 because only officers who had attained the rank of O-4 (Major or Lieutenant Commander) received enough retired pay to reach the ceiling. Less than 40 percent of retired officers had attained the O-4 rank (Report of The Subcommittee on Investigation of The House Committee on Post Office and Civil Service, 1978). Reserve officers and enlisted personnel were exempted from the statute. Subsequently regular officers retired for disability incurred in line of duty were also exempted.

The Depression-era Economy Act of 1932 placed a ceiling of $10,000 on the earnings of retired regular officers who were employed by the federal government. If total compensation exceeded $10,000, retired pay was to be reduced to maintain this level. Previous legislation disallowed employment if earnings exceeded a specified amount, but this statute permitted continued employment by placing a penalty on retired pay.

These statutes served to limit the employment alternatives of retired regular officers and denied the federal government the opportunity to employ retirees with specialized skills needed by the government. Throughout these years a central issue was whether or not an individual had a right to draw more than one check from the same underlying employer and if so should there be a limit to the amount of compensation that one should be eligible to receive. Powerful arguments are made on both sides of the issue. These were epitomized in the Dual Compensation Act of 1964 and the subsequent hearings to consider changes held by the Subcommittee on Investigations of the House Committee on Post Office and Civil Service, House of Representatives, Ninety-fifth Congress, First Session in 1977.

By 1963 there were over forty different laws and about two hundred separate Comptroller General decisions involving dual compensation matters (Report of The Subcommittee on Investigations of The House Committee on Post Office and Civil Service, 1977). The Dual Compensation Act of 1964 was an attempt to establish a comprehensive policy concerning the employment of retired military personnel in the federal civil service and the employment of civilians in more than one federal civil service position. Previous statutes were repealed and all provisions were codified into one law that would supposedly be easy to interpret and administer. It was to allow the government to recruit qualified retired military persons for hard-to-fill positions yet at the same time assure safeguards that would provide protection for federal civilian employees against unfair competition of retirees.

Attempts were made to include all retirees under the act, but it eventually evolved that only regular officers were affected, as had been the precedent historically. The act entitled retirees to the full salary of the civil service position for which they were employed, but it restricted the amount of retired pay to the first $2,000 plus 50 percent of any remaining amount. The $2,000 base was to be increased in accordance with the Consumer Price Index. In 1982 the base amount had increased to $6,529.39. Some exceptions were permitted in programs such as the space effort, for physicians, the President of the Senate, the Speaker of the House, and the Architect of the Capitol. Retirees were prohibited from employment in any Department of Defense activity for 180 days following retirement. Civilian employees argued that the 180-day delay was necessary to minimize the "buddy-system." Retirees argued that it was an unfair restriction and limited their job opportunities (Report of the Subcommittee on Investigations of The House Committee on Post Office and Civil Service, 1978).

Attention was again focused upon dual compensation in the early and middle 1970s. At this time the term "double-dipping" came into popular vogue and was espoused by President Carter who insisted upon legislative changes. Hearings were again held by the Subcommittee on Investigations of the House Committee on Post Office and Civil Service. Four main issues arose:

1. The simultaneous payment of both full uniformed services' retired pay and full federal civilian salary by the same underlying employer, the federal government.
2. The excepting of certain regular officers from the retired pay provisions of the Dual Compensation Act of 1964.
3. The extent to which retirees of the uniformed services may receive preferential treatment in obtaining federal civilian positions.
4. The desirability of employing retirees of the uniformed services in federal civilian positions (Report of The Subcommittee on Investigations of The House Committee on Post Office and Civil Service, 1977).

Although the above four issues surfaced repeatedly during the hearings, one received a disproportionate amount of attention, that dealing with the amount of money earned. Robert C. Nix, chairman of the subcommittee, in his introductory remarks opening the hearing, gave a flavor of the source of concern,

> The central issue thus far has been the payment of retired military pay together with full civilian salary. This is dramatically illustrated by this committee's findings that there may be as many as 10 retired flag rank military whose combined military pension and Federal civilian salary exceed the total salary paid the Vice President and Chief Justice of the Supreme Court and as many as 25 more who receive more than members of the President's Cabinet (Report of The Subcommittee on Investigations of The House Committee on Post Office and Civil Service, 1977).

Data utilized by Chairman Nix were compiled as of June 30, 1975. At that time there were 2.8 million federal civil servants and of this number slightly less than 142,000 were retired military personnel or about 5 percent of the total. The 142,000 represented approximately 14 percent of all retired military personnel. John Sheffey, executive vice president, National Association of Uniformed Services, responded to Chairman Nix,

> Let me treat now the small percentage of retired senior officers—colonels and generals—in the Civil Service . . . The total number at present is 177 Generals and Admirals and 2,500 Colonels, less than 2% of the 142,000 . . . These senior military retirees represent less than $\frac{1}{10}$ of 1% of the 2.8 million civilian employees of the Federal government (Report of The Subcommittee on Investigations of The House Committee on Post Office and Civil Service, 1977).

Most of the retirees are employed by the Department of Defense and the Post Office. Most of those employed in federal civil service jobs, as shown in Table 2.14, are enlisted personnel.

The impact of dual compensation is apparent in the total figures if the regular officer column is examined. Less than 4 percent of retired regular officers are employed in federal civil service. Over 75 percent of the employed retirees are

Table 2.14 Retirees in Federal Civil Service (Numbers by Rank and Component)

Commissioned officers	Regular	Nonregular	Total
O-10	16	0	16
O-9	34	0	34
0-8	45	22	67
O-7	39	21	60
O-6	1,061	1,425	2,486
O-5	1,347	7,334	8,681
O-4	770	6,702	7,472
O-3	492	1,979	2,471
O-2	241	1,175	1,416
O-1	55	339	394
Total	4,100	18,997	23,097
Warrant officers			
W-4	228	647	875
W-3	190	1,373	1,563
W-2	359	1,228	1,587
W-1	287	273	560
Total	1,064	3,521	4,585
Enlisted			
E-9			5,566
E-8			13,174
E-7			44,174
E-6			31,510
E-5			12,048
E-4			2,604
E-3			1,349
E-2			575
E-1			86
Total enlisted			111,793
Total unspecified			2,342
Total			141,817

Source: Report, *Dual Compensation Paid to Retired Uniformed Services' Personnel in Federal Civilian Positions,* 1977

enlisted personnel. The federal civil service represents a source of employment primarily then for enlisted personnel and nonregular officers.

Total compensation has been a key issue, as indicated previously. Table 2.15 gives the average total earnings for each rank level of retirees who were employed in the federal civil service system as of June 30, 1977.

Average total compensation exceeded $30,000 per year for less than 15 percent of all retirees. Most, in fact, had total compensation of less than $25,000 annually.

Favoritism in employment, or the so-called "buddy system," was examined during the hearings. It was concluded that favoritism is an elusive concept to concretize. Approximately ten complaints are filed each month, but fewer than 10 percent of these cases contain sufficient substantive evidence to warrant further investigation. Although in some situations the appearance of favoritism may have existed, documentation has not been possible generally. Several individuals believed if a buddy system did in fact exist, it would not be any different from that which exists in other settings.

There was general agreement that dual compensation was simply symptomatic of the basic problem—early retirement. As long as career military personnel can attain retirement eligibility after twenty years of active duty, they will need to seek second-career employment and the federal civil service is a potential source of employment. In a way the military retiree is a victim of the system in which he or she elected to make a career. It is of interest that the Post Office and Civil Service Committee held the hearings rather than the Armed Services Committee. Although impartiality should be exercised by either committee, the primary clientele of each would necessarily be different.

CONFLICT OF INTEREST

The first conflict of interest statute was enacted in 1896 and applied only to Navy officers, but a similar restriction was placed upon Army officers in 1923 that prevented retired officers from selling products or supplies to the military establishment (Hearings, *Employment of Retired Military and Civilian Personnel by Defense Industries,* 1959). There are five federal statutes that embody the conflict of interest legislation:

Table 2.15 Total Compensation: Retired Pay and Civil Service Salary for all Uniformed Service Retirees, June 30, 1977[a]

Rank at retirement	Number of retirees	Average retired pay	Average CS salary	Average total compensation
O-10	16	$39,046	$42,271	$81,317
O-9	34	37,790	45,503	83,293
O-8	67	28,508	40,514	69,022
O-7	60	22,816	38,132	60,948
O-6	2,486	17,667	30,902	48,569
O-5	8,681	13,058	23,658	36,569
O-4	7,472	10,450	20,163	30,613
O-3	2,471	8,786	18,478	27,263
O-2	1,416	6,903	18,487	25,390
O-1	394	5,880	18,811	24,691
Total commissioned officers	23,097	11,874	22,478	34,352
W-4	875	11,381	17,401	28,782
W-3	1,563	8,343	16,979	25,322
W-2	1,587	7,163	15,927	23,090
W-1	560	5,778	16,152	21,930
Total warrant officers	4,585	8,202	15,594	23,796
	27,682	11,265	21,336	32,601

Table 2.15, cont.

Total officers				
E-9	5,566	9,799	15,140	24,939
E-8	13,174	7,726	14,258	21,984
E-7	44,881	6,149	14,059	20,208
E-6	31,510	5,222	12,778	18,000
E-5	12,048	4,378	12,261	16,639
E-4	2,604	3,949	12,679	16,628
E-3	1,349	3,789	13,284	17,073
E-2	575	3,731	13,490	17,221
E-1	86	3,007	12,640	15,647
Total enlisted	111,793	5,970	13,557	19,527
Total	139,475	7,020	15,100	22,120

[a]The average retired pay and civil service salaries for those retirees in ranks 0-10 through 0-6 are based on those retirees employed on a full-time basis.

Source: Report, *Dual Compensation Paid to Retired Uniformed Services Personnel,* 1978

1. Title 18, United States Code, Section 207. This is referred to as the Ethics in Government Act and prohibits all retired officers and former civilian personnel from "switching sides" in matters previously under their control or cognizance while in government service.
2. Title 18, United States Code 281. The so-called "criminal selling statute" that imposes a lifetime prohibition on retired regular officers representing any person in the sale of anything to the branch of service in which the officer holds his retired status.
3. Title 18, United States Code 283. Prohibits retired regular officers from prosecuting claims against the government within two years of their retirement.
4. Title 37, United States Code 801 "C". Prohibits the payment of retired pay to any regular officer engaged in selling "supplies or war materials" to any of the uniformed services within three years of retirement.
5. Title 50, United States Code 1436, is a registration statute. It requires all GS-14s and O-4s and above to register for three years following retirement if they are employed by a defense contractor who does over $10 million business with the government or is paying the retiree $15,000 or more in salary (Taussig, 1981).

Many officers feel very strongly about the conflict of interest legislation. They believe it interferes with their quest for employment and impugns their integrity (McNeil, 1964).

Persuasive arguments can be made for the need for both conflict of interest and dual compensation laws; however, their effect is to pose an economic restriction on the retiree, with the greatest impact upon the retired regular officer.

3

SOCIOLOGICAL DILEMMAS OF MILITARY RETIREMENT

Introduction

The military retirement system has for many years been a major public policy concern, in part, because of its increasing costs. In 1956, for example, this country expended over $500 million on retired military personnel. By 1980 expenditures for military retirement totaled more than $11 billion—twenty times more than the amount expended in 1956 (Cooper, 1981). Furthermore, the cost of retired pay is increasing disproportionately so that by the year 2020, expenditures for retired pay are expected to be as much as 30 percent of the total budget for military personnel (Biderman, 1971).

In addition to these dramatic cost increases, the effectiveness of military retirement policy is being seriously questioned (*Report of the President's Commission on Military Compensation*, 1978). For example, the cost structure and operation of the military retirement system constitutes a special policy problem because the monies needed for maintaining the system must be appropriated anew each year. Unlike many other pension systems, the military retirement system is noncontributory, nonfunded, nonvested, and noninvested. As a result the annual appropriation character of the system gives it special and painful political visibility (Biderman, 1973). It is clear, as noted by Cooper, "that some revision of the present system is warranted, but any examination of that system, or of the possible alternatives to it, must include consideration of many different issues" (R. Cooper, 1981).

The tendency in the general population is to equate retirement with aging, reduced income owing to unemployment or drastically reduced labor force participation, dependency, and constructive use of leisure time (McNeil, 1976). Much has been written about the problems and prospects of occupational retirement within the general population. Very little however, has been written about retired military personnel who, because of their occupational choice, have retired from active duty at a relatively earlier age (e.g., the average age at retirement for career military personnel, excluding nondisability retirees, is about forty-five). As mentioned before, military retirement is based upon a length of service principle, in contrast to age plus length of service in other occupational groups. Current law allows career military personnel to retire after twenty years of active duty. As a result, the retired military population differs markedly from other retired population groups in such key respects as age and physical health. Retirement, therefore, has a special meaning for the career military man and his family that differs from those in other occupations.

Military retirement can be studied from several important perspectives: 1. its impact upon the military establishment, 2. its impact upon the military retiree and his family, and 3. its impact upon society. The focus of this chapter will be upon the impact of military retirement on the retiree and his family and the effects of retirement upon society.

Descriptive Characteristics of the Retired Military Population

Unlike most retirement systems, military retirement uses the criteria of length of service and physical condition rather than age as the primary determinant of retirement (Biderman, 1959).

This means that military retirees, in most cases, are far younger at time of retirement than their civilian counterparts. A recent compilation of data on age at time of retirement for military personnel gave the average age as forty-three years old for officers and thirty-nine years old for enlisted personnel (Defense Manpower Data Center, 1981b). Most retirees are likely also to be married and the parents of two or three school-age children (McNeil and Giffen, 1965a).

Those who retire upon achieving twenty years of service will retire with remuneration amounting to somewhat less than half their earnings prior to retirement. The retiree from active duty receives an immediate annuity calculated at 2.5 percent of base pay for each year of creditable service, subject to a maximum of 75 percent of base pay. Base pay is "equal to final basic pay if the retiree first became a member of the Armed Services before Sept. 8th, 1980. For those new members after that date, base pay equals the average of the highest 36 months of pay" (Defense Manpower Data Center, 1981b). In calculating years of service, over six months service is rounded up to a full year. Additionally, a member of the military has no vested right in the retirement system until the point of retirement eligibility.

In fiscal year 1980, there were 1.1 million retired, nondisability annuitants (who were paid $10.5 billion), 200,000 disability annuitants (who were paid $1.2 billion), and 67,000 survivor benefit families (who received $256 million) in the military retirement system. The average gross retirement pay of nondisability retired officers was $1,676 per month and nondisabled enlistees averaged $728 per month (Valuation of the Military Retirement System, FY 1980). While seemingly substantial, the gross monthly retirement pay of most retirees will be insufficient to support their families at their accustomed standard of living (Biderman, 1959; McNeil and Giffen, 1965a; 1965b). As a result, many retirees need to work and supplement their retirement pensions by working in the civilian labor market. The need to work is further heightened by the fact that many retirees have family responsibilities and an emotional need to maintain gainful employment in some type of productive work. The average number of dependents of military personnel with between twenty and thirty years of service is slightly over three (Biderman, 1964). A majority of the retirees' dependents are children who are in the costly years of secondary school or college.

The emotional need to work is epitomized by the status losses and role conflicts that retirees experience when they exchange the uniforms for civilian clothes. Whatever civilian activities the retiree elects to engage in, he/she probably must begin at or near the bottom of the hierarchic ladder (McNeil and Giffen, 1965b). Often, this loss of status is a traumatic experience not only for the retiree but for his family who are subject to a loss of prestige derived from the retiree's previous military occupation.

Several researchers have identified particular problems faced by military retirees either before or following their retirement from active duty (McNeil and Giffen, 1965a; 1965b; 1967). The transition from military life to civilian life can lead to a constellation of symptoms, which have been called the "retirement syndrome" (McNeil and Giffen, 1967). These symptoms include anxiety, irritability, apathy, increased alcohol use, depression, somatic complaints, role confusion, and family and/or marital discord. As noted by Wolpert:

> The significance of these symtoms with respect to the adequate adjustment of the retiree can be serious and long term. Contributing to the syndrome appear to be feelings in the retiree of not being useful coupled with loss of the prestige, problems in the direct translation of military occupations into a civilian counterpart, and difficulty accepting and being accepted by the civilian environment (Wolpert, et al., 1982).

Additionally, all military retirees go through a period of role confusion or conflict. Retirees, having attained some measure of social stuatus, role identification, and responsibility during their time in the armed services, must now adapt and adjust to life in the civilian world. In general, they have no specific or identifiable roles and must now establish new patterns of behavior, interaction, and functioning if they are to be successfully integrated into mainstream civilian life. Most retirees undoubtedly negotiate this period of change without much difficulty and make a relatively good adjustment to their environment; others, however, may need the services of trained professionals in order to make satisfactory adjustments to the requirements of civilian life.

Problems may also arise when retirees attempt to secure employment in the labor market. The period in which the retiree spends seeking suitable employment can be an agonizing time, with the retiree experiencing varying emotional states and levels of activity. McNeil (1976) identifies four distinct phases that retirees go through in search of appropriate employment. He stated:

> Initially there appears to be a period of optimism accompanied by considerable job-hunting activity. During this phase, the retiree tends to view other similarly unemployed retirees as persons who are not really serious about working and, therefore, have not vigorously sought work, believing that anyone who wants a job can find a job. . . . In the second stage, practically all leads, potential leads, or even hints of leads may be pursued. Activity of this nature is reflected by increased anxiety which frequently represents wasted effort and energy. The effects of repeated rejections begin to take a toll. In the third phase, the retiree begins to doubt his worth and employability and spends fewer hours in job seeking activity. . . . During the fourth phase, there is often a reduction in job expectations, and the retiree makes a more realistic appraisal of such factors as the potential labor market in his locale. He is more willing to lower his salary minimum and is more frequently inclined to accept employment in geographic areas that were his second or third choices in terms of desireability. . . . In some ways the retiree's morale is at a new low, the financial situation may be critical or approaching desperation, and familial pressure is at a new high.

Thus, age, familial responsibility, social pressure, and the material and emotional need to work force the retired serviceman to seek employment. This process however, can be anxiety-producing and frustrating not only for the retiree but for each member in his family. The time immediately subsequent to retirement has the potential for being emotionally distressing for all family members (McNeil, 1976). Each member experiences some degree of stress as the family attempts to adjust to retired life.

Socio-Psychological Determinants of Retirement

Military administrative policies may require involuntary retirement for varied reasons, such as age, disability, reductions in personnel levels, or to create promotional opportunities for younger active duty employees. Retirement may also occur voluntarily for many reasons. In the first instance, the individual has no choice in the retirement decision, and retirement is often seen in a negative light by the retiree. The military system with its emphasis on youthful vigor and a continual need for changing skills must thrust most career personnel out of the system at an early age. Most retirees are forced out of the armed forces at, or shortly after, they have served twenty years, and practically all are retired before they have exceeded thirty years of service (Biderman, 1973).

Career military personnel who retire voluntarily also do so for many reasons. In a recent survey by the Department of Defense, many retirees cited several influences on their decision to retire (*Military Retiree Survey Report,* 1978). Table 3.1 identifies major influences on the decision to retire among officers and enlisted personnel. Officers and enlisted personnel cited similar influences on their voluntary decisions to retire. A majority of the enlisted men and almost half of the officers stated that they wanted to seek employment (a second career) in the civilian labor market. The possibility of an undesirable assignment was not as important to officers (18.4 percent) as it was to enlisted men (32.1 percent) in influencing their retirement decision. Both groups responded similarly regarding poor promotion possibilities and the failure to be promoted as important determinants of their retirement decisions.

Table 3.1 Major Influences on Decision to Retire

Major influences	Percent of respondents per influence	
	Officers	Enlisted
Wanted second career	44.6	56.6
Possibility of undesirable assignments	18.4	32.1
Failed to be promoted	24.9	28.5
Poor promotion possibilities	21.4	35.1

Source: Military Retiree Survey Report, 1978

Age is also an important factor in most decisionmaking involving retirement. As has been mentioned, most military retirees seek employment in civilian labor markets following retirement. Employment choices, however, become more and more limited the older the retiree is at the time he/she seeks employment. Many prospective retirees plan for retirement by the time they are in their early forties because of the tendency for most civilian industries to place a premium on these age levels for hiring new employees. McNeil cogently notes that "age, again becomes critical relative to family pressure. High school age children are very resistant to changing schools and not being able to graduate with their classmates. Wives are often ready to secure a home and become established in a community. Familial pressure at this time in life may precipitate the decision to retire, should reassignment to another military installation be required" (McNeil, 1976).

Some individuals retire from active duty because of disagreement with military policy. Such individuals handle their disagreements by exercising their option to initiate action for voluntary retirement. Still others initiate retirement actions because they perceive limited or no opportunity for promotion or advancement. This group would include persons who feel they have not attained the rank they expected and those who have been promoted to the top of their heirarchy but are still ambitious and motivated to get ahead and cannot tolerate being stymied (i.e., noncommissioned officers who have been promoted to pay grade E-9 or officers who are colonels and see little opportunity for being elevated to general). It is of interest that factors influencing the retirement decision are, for the most part, situations that career service persons accept as a necessary part of military life. Once retirement eligibility has been attained, these formerly accepted conditions become intolerable irritants that influence the decision to retire.

Financial and economic gain has also been a factor influencing many to retire from active service. An active duty person who has a transferrable skill that brings a lucrative salary in the civilian labor market might be inclined to retire from active duty at, or shortly after, twenty years. A retirement pension coupled with a relatively high salary from a civilian job may place some retirees at a considerably higher income level than that received while on active duty. Thus, under these circumstances, the incentive to retire is very high indeed.

Labor Force Participation: Second Careers of Military Retirees

Although military retired pay provides a significant financial base for most retirees, particularly those who retire as officers of relatively high rank, they still must supplement their incomes by working in the civilian labor market. Moreover, even if there are no pressing financial needs or obligations, most retirees feel that they are too young to retire in the conventional sense, that is, to a life of unrelieved leisure. Consequently, the meaning of retirement in its "traditional sense of leaving remunerative employment will hardly be applicable [or descriptive of] to the large majority of the retired military population at any time in the foreseeable future" (Biderman, 1965, p. 295). Hence, despite the comparative generosity of the military retirement program, it does not adequately fulfill the economic needs of most retirees nor is retired pay seen as the sole or major source of income. Retired persons must take on civilian employment if an appreciable reduction in income is to be avoided. Additionally, social and psychological factors require almost all retirees to continue working until conventional retirement (e.g., for most occupational groups this is sixty-five to seventy years of age).

The military personnel structure depends upon the majority of its members being forced to leave the service at ages (mid-forties) regarded as the middle of the work life and be able to obtain civilian employment comparable to their military status (Biderman and Sharp, 1968). Evidence from studies indicate that generally most retirees have obtained jobs (Cooper, 1981; Biderman, 1964; 1959; Military Retiree Survey Report, 1978). Despite the large number of studies that have been conducted, it is not possible to give a satisfactory answer to the question, "How well off is the retired serviceman compared to his situation in the service?" Biderman, in his study of the retired military, suggests that retiree post-retirement income, including retired pay, is at least roughly equal to the total emoluments of active duty (Biderman, 1971). Analyzing data from the 1977 DOD retiree survey, Cooper indicates that military retirees fare better in their post-service (second career) earnings and employment than previous studies have indicated (Cooper, 1981). For example, data in Table 3.2 shows that retired officers' wages and salary earnings in 1976 averaged $12,168, about 25 percent below those of nonretiree veterans; enlisted retirees' 1976 average wage and salary earnings averaged $10,142, only about 15 percent below those of comparably aged and educated nonretiree veterans. The differences between the groups are almost entirely accounted for by the fact that military retirees worked fewer hours and/or weeks than nonretirees. Table 3.2 also indicates that officer and enlisted retirees working full-time, year-round earned about the same, on the average, as nonretirees who worked full-time, year-round.

The post-retirement incomes revealed by surveys of the military suggest that the assumptions underlying the second-career retirement system have worked out satisfactorily. The majority of the men leaving the services because of retirement have obtained employment that in combination with their

Table 3.2 Military Retirees' and Nonretirees' Average Post-Service Earnings in 1976

	Military Retirees					Nonretirees	
Sample	Retired 0-3 yrs.	Retired 4-7 yrs.	Retired 8-11 yrs.	Retired 12 yrs.	All	Veterans	Nonveterans
All							
Officer	$ 9,547	$10,826	$13,262	$13,505	$12,168	$16,179	$14,274
Enlisted	6,919	9,903	11,771	10,660	10,142	12,083	10,892
Full time, year round employed							
Officer	16,222	17,712	18,848	19,820	18,650	18,284	16,513
Enlisted	11,447	12,661	14,427	14,177	13,521	14,300	12,758

Source: R. V. L. Cooper, 1981

pension benefits, have allowed them to somewhat maintain their accustomed standard of living. However, it is quite possible that future retirees may experience severe economic hardship after retirement because of higher rates of unemployment and periods of labor surplus.

In 1977, 25 percent of retired officers and more than 15 percent of enlisted men were not working and not looking for work, going to school, and/or voluntarily working part-time (R.V.L. Cooper, 1981). Either retirees take a considerable period of time to reach full earning potential or more recent retirees have less civilian job potential (Biderman, 1971). A similar conclusion is suggested by Cooper's analysis of DOD data. He indicates that the vast majority of retirees who seek post-service employment find it in a relatively short time period (e.g., 90 percent of all retirees find a job within six months or less), although, in many cases, they are forced to accept a lower wage initially in order to secure this employment (R.V.L. Cooper, 1981). Even those retirees employed full-time, year-round receive lower annual earnings during their first few post-retirement years. For example, fully employed retired officers earned about $35,000 less during the three to six-year transistion period than they would if there were no such transition; fully employed enlisted retirees earn about $20,000 less than their nonretiree counterparts (R.V.L. Cooper, 1981). Thus, although military retirees eventually fare quite well relative to their nonretired peers, there is a transition period during which their earnings are substantially less.

In 1982, approximately 11 percent of the labor force in this country was unemployed. Automation and technological advances in many industrial areas have meant that more and more workers will be replaced by machines that are more efficient and effective. As a result, future military retirees will be entering a rapidly shrinking labor market and will find themselves in severe competition with civilians for a limited number of jobs. Since the retirees are veterans, they will be entitled to special consideration if they seek federal civil service positions. Moreover, many retirees, by receiving retired pay, may be willing to compete for specific jobs at lower salaries than most civilians would be willing to accept. Thus, military retirees may find themselves in the position of adversely affecting prevailing wage rates (McNeil, 1965b; Biderman, 1971; 1973).

The potential impact of large-scale military retirement on the labor market becomes clearer when we analyze geographical patterns relating to retirement residences. Approximately 20 percent of retirees settle in California, and slightly less than 10 percent in Texas and Florida respectively. Similarly, approximately 10 percent reside in the Virginia-Maryland-District of Columbia areas. New York and Washington, with about 5 percent respectively, are also popular residential areas. The retiree's choice of an area to settle in is influenced by such factors as its proximity to large permanent military installations, the availability and quality of hospitals, recreation, exchange and commissary facilities, the desireability of the climate, and the availability of employment opportunities (McNeil, 1976; Biderman, 1971). Most retirees establish themselves reasonably close to a military post because of the important retirement benefits, such as commissaries and medical facilities, that are available there. Just commissary and post exchange privileges can be worth six to seven hundred dollars (in 1982 dollars this figure is approximately $1,200) per year for a family of four (Biderman, 1971). Since retirees do not settle at random throughout a state but tend to cluster in specific areas (i.e., San Antonio, Texas; Phoenix, Arizona; Colorado Springs and Denver, Colorado; Montgomery, Alabama; Seattle, Washington, etc.), they are likely to affect the labor markets in these areas. One effect of this concentration will be competition for jobs among the retirees and other groups. The entrance into the civilian labor force of selected communities by large numbers of retirees, for whom it may be feasible to accept employment at rates of remuneration below that for persons of comparable status, is a development some will see as a threat (Biderman, 1959).

Future studies of the impact of retiree concentration and the specific impact of these retirees on the labor market will, hopefully, provide more insight and understanding as well as

Table 3.3 Residence of Military Retirees by State for Fiscal Year 1981 and 1982

State	1980	1981	Increase	Percent increase
Alabama	28,997	29,711	714	2.5
Alaska	3,770	3,933	163	4.3
Arizona	27,782	28,656	874	3.1
Arkansas	16,967	17,274	307	1.8
California	190,593	194,871	4,278	2.2
Colorado	29,348	30,043	695	2.4
Connecticut	9,530	9,630	100	1.0
Delaware	3,805	3,855	50	1.3
D. of Columbia	5,124	4,911	−213	−4.2
Florida	111,343	113,917	2,574	2.3
Georgia	43,703	44,756	1,053	2.4
Guam/Agana	460	459	−1	−0.2
Hawaii	9,040	9,156	116	1.3
Idaho	5,707	5,913	206	3.6
Illinois	23,388	23,575	187	0.8
Indiana	13,662	13,916	254	1.9
Iowa	6,334	6,472	138	2.2
Kansas	12,543	12,826	283	2.3
Kentucky	15,117	15,197	80	0.5
Louisiana	21,537	22,136	599	2.8
Maine	7,333	7,516	183	2.5
Maryland	29,206	29,717	511	1.7
Massachusetts	19,905	19,948	43	0.2
Michigan	16,893	16,946	53	0.3
Minnesota	9,821	10,071	250	2.5
Mississippi	15,891	16,181	290	1.8
Missouri	21,669	22,059	390	1.8

some definitive answers to those most concerned about these issues. Table 3.3 indicates the retirement residences of military retirees by states. Examination of the states of residence and the percentage increases reaffirms the preferences of retirees for warmer climate areas. At the same time, however, there appears to be a relatively large percentage increase in cold climate states such as Alaska, Idaho, South Dakota, Vermont, and Wyoming.

The transferability of military skills to civilian jobs is also a matter of immense concern to both retirees and the military

Table 3.3, cont.

Montana	3,799	3,901	102	2.7
Nebraska	7,373	7,514	141	1.9
Nevada	10,386	10,889	503	4.8
New Hampshire	6,597	6,752	155	2.3
New Jersey	21,862	21,810	−52	−0.2
New Mexico	11,899	12,265	366	3.1
New York	33,394	33,995	601	1.8
North Carolina	37,968	39,061	1,093	2.9
North Dakota	1,608	1,670	62	3.9
Ohio	26,529	26,799	270	1.0
Oklahoma	22,010	22,722	712	3.2
Oregon	14,420	14,833	413	2.9
Pennsylvania	33,048	33,492	444	1.3
Puerto Rico	5,220	5,489	269	5.2
Rhode Island	5,465	5,456	−9	−0.2
South Carolina	30,789	31,516	727	2.4
South Dakota	2,420	2,497	77	3.2
Tennessee	25,379	25,966	587	2.3
Texas	112,799	116,359	3,560	3.2
Utah	5,900	6,226	326	5.5
Vermont	2,026	2,062	36	1.8
Virginia	68,250	69,626	1,376	2.0
Virgin Islands	147	205	58	39.5
Washington	42,499	44,030	1,531	3.6
West Virginia	6,850	6,994	144	2.1
Wisconsin	9,855	10,043	188	1.9
Wyoming	2,349	2,438	89	3.8
Other	14,216	10,707	−3,509	−24.7
Total	1,264,525	1,288,962	24,437	1.9

Source: Defense Manpower Data Center, 1981

personnel structure, which depends upon the majority of its members being able to find civilian employment comparable to their military status. The actual degree to which retirees use their military acquired skills in their civilian jobs is difficult to assess. Sharp and Biderman (1966) indicate that close relationships between military and second-career occupational specialities occurred only in a minority of those they surveyed. Such relationships obtain more often for enlisted men than for officers, but even among enlisted men, close correspondence between military speciality and civilian job was far from universal. Biderman and Sharp, in a later study of the transferability of military skills state:

> The transfer from military to civilian occupations took place without much formal retraining, although those who did undergo training fared better, and a substantial number expressed a need for further training. Apparently, general qualifications—education, in particular—rather than highly specific technical skills were the most frequent bases for obtaining work. Success in the civilian job market was positively related to various indexes of success and integration with the military, rather than with military marginality (Biderman and Sharp, 1968).

Thus, it appears that educational attainment is the most significant correlate of second-career success. Moreover, in analyzing the considerations that entered into employers' evaluations of retiree's job qualification, Biderman and Sharp (1968) found that various criteria such as the retiree's ability to articulate, personality characteristics, and status (i.e., rank achieved during military duty) were given uppermost consideration. In addition, they found that in both hiring and assigning men, employers usually did not attempt specific matching of jobs and specific military acquired skills. In all likelihood, the transferability of military skills in general is less of a problem than it is usually thought to be. Retirees who were successful in the military establishment tended to be most successful in their civilian job-seeking efforts and second careers. Second-career jobs obtained by retired military personnel show very high association between civilian income and job satisfaction on the one hand and success in the military career on the other (Biderman and Sharp, 1968; Biderman, 1971).

The Impact of Military Retirement on Social and Political Institutions

As large numbers of military retirees congregate in many local communities, one question that arises is to what extent will they utilize social institutions and influence political processes? Existing studies of military retirement are, for a variety of reasons, unable to provide us with definitive answers to this important question. To date, there is limited information on how the retired integrate themselves into the communities in which they reside, the extent to which they are involved in political activities and processes, and the degree to which they utilize community resources. An early study by Watson (1963) suggests that most military retirees attempt to maintain continued psychological identification with the military institution (e.g., they continue to read military literature, desire close contact with nearby military installations, discuss military affairs with friends, etc.). Watson, in turn, further suggests that these ties do not interfere with the retiree's abilities to integrate into civilian communities but, in most cases, they appear to facilitate it. For many retirees, integration into local communities is made easier because many of the skills they acquired in military life (i.e., exercising authority, making oral presentations, participating in organized meetings, etc.) have value in community leadership positions.

Because of their leadership skills, many retirees (especially retired officers) tend to be very active and influential in community social agencies and other organizations. They disproportionately gravitate toward leadership positions in voluntary associations, both those of a distinctive character like Retired Officers Associations and veterans organizations, and those of more general character such as political, business, and human service organizations (Biderman, 1959).

Since most retirees do, in fact, work full-time and year-round, the time available to them to pursue social and political interest is limited. As a consequence, it is unlikely that large numbers of them in any particular community will be interested in pursuing activities to gain control of a community's social and/or political institutions. McNeil, in a commentary relative to this issue notes:

> At present, it is doubtful that military retirees exert any appreciable political influence in local communities. Occasionally

a military retiree reaches a position of political prominence [e.g., witness Alexander Haig's rise to political prominence], but such persons appear to be the exception rather than the rule (McNeil, 1965b).

Thus, retirees as a group have not constituted a significant social or political force. Political activities by retiree organizations has been limited largely to matters of direct material concern, such as retired pay legislation (Biderman, 1973). There appears to be important carry over of the doctrine of a political neutrality from active duty to the retired status. Available evidence, however, strongly suggests that retirees as a group are neither more active nor more lethargic than other citizen groups in engaging in social and political processes. An important question that remains to be answered in assessing the social and political influences of retirees is the actual degree of homogeneity and concert of this population, that is, are they a homogeneous group in terms of interests and ideologies? (Biderman, 1973)

Military Retirement and the Family: A Scenario

The military establishment can be conceptualized as a distinct social system that dramatically influences the patterns of values and behaviors of its members and their families (McNeil and Giffen, 1967; McNeil, 1976; Frances and Gale, 1973). Few professional or occupational groups have work and nonwork roles and activities as interdependent as those found in the military. As a result, there is little loss of identity between work roles and home life. This tends to be more so if the family occupies a residence on a military installation. Social and recreational activities of the family tend to be heavily centered around interactions with other military families and, in many instances, exclude contacts with nonmilitary ones. Health, social, and welfare services are provided within the confines of the military community, making it unnecessary to seek services in the civilian community. Examples of these resources are "Officers and Noncommissioned officers clubs, with their wives' activities that center around swimming pools, riding stables, bowling alleys, and even aeroclubs" (McNeil, 1976). Schools, nurseries, hospitals, chapels, and commissaries may also be provided.

Such environments, however, can produce serious stresses for military families. Since families reside, work, and attend school in a tightly organized community that demands conformity to many norms and values, acceptable behaviors of family members are predetermined (Frances and Gale, 1973). As a result, there is low tolerance for individual variations in behavior. Shame and fear of ostracism by those outside the family may encourage scapegoating within the family.

During the past several decades there has been some breakdown in the extent of social cohesiveness within the military community. Since World World II, it has been necessary to maintain a relatively large military force that, for the most part, has been manned largely by short-term personnel who remain primarily civilian-oriented. The general increase in numbers and types of people within the military community has presented formidable policy problems. In the area of housing, for example, McNeil notes: "Sufficient family housing on the military installation is not available to provide a residence for each family. Large numbers of families live in the civilian community, thus increasing the demarcation between work and social roles" (McNeil, 1976).

Additionally, recent studies have shown that because of its culture and social structure, the military establishment has created serious inequities in the responsiveness of its social welfare and health provision to the needs of individuals and families within it and those making transitions from it (Maynard and Blalock, 1977; Ayers, 1977).

As shown elsewhere, many military retirees seek employment in the civilian labor market for a variety of reasons. Many of them have experienced periods of unemployment and have often needed to take jobs that were not equivalent to the skill level and prestige of their former military position (e.g., oftentimes earnings from civilian jobs, when combined with retired pay, may just equal, or be less, than previously received military pay). Status mobility in a downward direction may precipitate stress not only for the the retireee but his family as well. In commenting on this issue, Bernard notes: "Even if the man himself does not break under the loss of status in downward mobility, his family may become a casualty. The man may lose face with his wife and children. They may cease to respect him, or even worse, come to pity or condemn him" (Bernard, 1957).

A 1976 study conducted by Platte confirmed, in part, Bernard's hypothesis. Platte's study was directed toward ascertaining whether or not there were significant differences in the level of psychological well-being and/or marital adjustment among three socially mobile groups of military retirees (upward, horizontal, downward). He found that the direction of perceived social mobility made a difference in the levels of psychological well-being for retired officers, retired enlisted men, and the wives of retired enlisted men. However, perceptions of social mobility did not appear to have an effect on the psychological well-being of the wives of retired officers. Additionally, the overall interpretation of his data suggested that the direction of perceived social mobility did make a difference in marital adjustment following military retirement. Platte states that

> horizontally mobile did not report significantly higher levels of marital adjustment than the vertically mobile. Nor did the upwardly mobile report significantly higher levels of marital adjustment than downwardly mobile retired officers. The noteworthy differences was between the unemployed officers and the downwardly mobile officers; unemployed officers are better adjusted in their marriages than downwardly mobile officers. The findings also indicated that perceived social mobility makes a difference in the marital adjustment of retired enlisted men, but the exact locations of these differences could not be specified (Platte, 1976).

Many retirees have returned to academic institutions for retraining in fields in which they may not have extensive prior knowledge or experience and in which they are in competition with much younger students with more current backgrounds (Maynard and Blalock, 1977). These transition experiences for retirees and their families can represent genuine life crises with resultant disruptions of emotional equilibrium and marital discord. Such turmoil and tensions may pervade the entire family structure and causally precipitate adverse reactions among all family members.

At or before the time of retirement from active duty, there may be concern by the family about the retiree's ability to compete successfully for meaningful jobs in the civilian labor market. The loss of security that was once provided by the military career may produce anxieties for the entire family. The intensity of these anxieties may range from minor expressions of concern about the impending adjustments that will be required to rather severe disabling psychic symptoms such as depression, apprehension, apathy, somatic complaints, acting out behavior in children, etc. (McNeil, 1976).

The transition for many retirees from a military environment to a civilian one occurs at a time when many of their wives are in a relatively vulnerable position with the onset of menopause and the resultant physiological problems to which they must also adjust (McNeil and Giffen, 1967). Characteristic stresses and previous coping mechanisms may not be very useful at this time. Wives who have developed successful coping devices in the past, however, probably will be less likely to be overwhelmed by retirement and its accompanying problems.

Retirement from active duty can represent a time of crisis for the retirees as well as their families. Individual family members may respond to crisis in a myriad of ways; some evidence a greater degree of disequilibrium than others. For most retirees and their families, however, the level of disequilibrium is probably minimal. Even among families who perceive retirement as an emotional threat, most will eventually make a relatively adequate adjustment to the normative requirements of civilian life. Retirees as well as their families, however, need to know what to expect during the pre- and post-retirement periods. The more information and understanding they have about retirement experiences, the better they will be able to cope with possible adverse effects. Adequate and systematic preretirement preparatory policies will be of immense benefit in minimizing transitional problems associated with military retirement.

Conclusions

The focus of this chapter has been on examining the sociological impacts of military retirement upon retirees, their families, and society. The armed services have only gradually began to give attention to the problems of military retirement. This change has been in response to an increase in the size of the retired population from an estimated 3,000 in the year 1900 (Giffen and McNeil, 1967) to nearly 60,000 new retirees throughout the 1980s. Generally, the lower age limit of retired populations studied is around sixty-five years, the traditional retirement age in this country. However, variants of this pattern have been emerging and military careerists are seen as a special group that merits attention as a data source for much needed information on early retirement and second careers (Platte, 1976).

There seems to be a consensus about the manifest institutional functions of the retirement system in the military. These include, among other things, maintaining a rank distribution that is approximately pyramidal in shape, keeping the opportunity system open for upward mobility within the organization, and providing a relatively young and healthy pool of human resources for carrying out defense activities (McNeil and Giffen, 1965b; Biderman and Sharp, 1968; Platte, 1976). Consequently, most active duty career personnel choose to retire shortly after twenty years rather than pursuing a full thirty-year career. From an individual standpoint, the vast majority of careerists are eligible to and do retire during what are seen as years of peak productivity.

In general, retirement benefits after twenty years of service include a minimum monthly retirement pay equivalent to 50 percent of basic pay at the time of separation. The limitations of retirement pay as the sole source of income, the relative youth of the retiree and his family, and the normatively prescribed value of work in our society are important factors that influence a vast majority of military retirees to seek employment in the civilian occupational structure (Biderman, 1971). Several seminal research studies have drawn the attention of decisionmakers, among others, to potentially problematic aspects of second career efforts and outcomes (Cooper, 1981; Biderman, 1971; Biderman and Sharp, 1968). However, few studies exist that have attempted to examine the ramifications of military retirement on retirees' personal identities, the psychological well-being of retirees and their families, and on social, political, and environmental institutions (McNeil and Giffen, 1965b; 1967; McNeil, 1976; Biderman, 1959). The data for these studies, however, have been derived principally from clinical populations. As a result, they fall short of representing the general population of retirees because of their methodological weaknesses, such as ex post facto designs and sampling bias. The inferences we can draw from these studies can only offer hypotheses to be subjected to scientific scrutiny rather than empirically supported theoretical assertions.

Despite their weaknesses, however, most of the studies of military retirement unquestionably contribute to improving our understanding of the retirement system's impact upon retirees, their families, and society by offering data upon which hypotheses can be formulated for more rigorous research and for more differentiated approaches to the study of retirees and their families (McCubbin, et al., 1976). As studies of the military retirement system move from observation and speculation to hypothesis testing designs, it is expected that we will not witness the independent amassing of simplistic data that does not take into account the wisdom of what has already been done. Rather, we expect that these studies will sensitize and influence policy makers to the immediate and long-range implications of their decisions affecting the retirement system, its ultimate impact on retirees and their families, and its impact on social institutions.

4

MENTAL HEALTH DILEMMAS OF MILITARY RETIREMENT

The Symbolic Meaning of Retirement

Individuals who have studied and written about the mental health impact of retirement upon the career military person seem to agree that retirement is significantly different for military careerists than it is for persons in other occupations. Much of this difference is related to the usual meaning of retirement and the nature of the military service. One significant variable, age, permeates the entire mental health issue of military retirement.

Retirement usually means a cessation of paid employment and a withdrawal from the work force. In most occupations retirement is not considered until the individual is sixty-five years of age or older. In fact, age sixty-five is considered the normal age for retirement and retirement before that is labeled "early" retirement. Use of the qualifying adjective suggests an atypical or unusual action. For the nonmilitary occupational groups, retirement means reduced income, removal from active paid full-time employment, and the constructive use of leisure time. The individual who retires at age sixty-five is visualized as one who has made his or her major contribution to society and is now entitled to a well-deserved life of leisure. The primary task facing the retiree is to adjust to the nonwork role. This transition is deemed to be a natural one associated with the slower physiological processes caused by aging. Retirees are expected to have minimal familial responsibility and reduced financial commitments. This idyllic symbolism of retirement is in marked contrast to what confronts the military retiree.

As one reviews the symbolic meanings of retirement, it becomes apparent that military retirement is markedly different from retirement in other occupational groups; the main difference primarily is age at the time of retirement. The only exceptions to this are in the other two hazardous occupational groups, police and fire department personnel. Military retirement is based upon a length of service principle and current law allows career armed forces personnel to retire after twenty years of active duty in the uniformed service. Since individuals may enlist as early as age seventeen, simple arithmetic indicates that a career military person may retire at age thirty-seven after having served twenty years. Retirement eligibility is reached before age forty-five for most career military personnel, and most career military personnel retire upon attaining retirement eligibility or soon thereafter.

At a time when most workers are in the midst of their peak years of earnings and productivity, the career military person is retiring. In a sense this may be seen as changing horses in the middle of the stream since military retirees usually seek full-time employment and do not retire to leisure. Because of family responsibility, work is necessary to maintain an accustomed standard of living. The typical retiree, at the time of retirement, has a spouse and two or three dependent school-age children. Retired pay varies from about 35 percent to 70 percent of gross active duty pay depending upon rank, years of military service, and special or incentive payments.

Contrary to public belief, few military retirees make a lateral or upgraded transfer to lucrative civilian employment. Often earnings from a civilian job combined with retired may just equal or be slightly more than previously received gross military pay. Employment is a necessity for economic as well as societal and personal needs. Our culture insists that able-bodied, middle-aged males be constructively employed, and most males do in fact feel an emotional need to work. This need to work, however, poses special problems for the military retiree. Because of the years spent in the military service, the retiree may be at a competitive disadvantage due to transferability of skills problems and knowing how to sell one's skills in a nonmilitary job market. These factors combine to increase the likelihood that the military retiree will have difficulty securing suitable employment and that the employment secured will be at a level below the responsibility and authority attained in the military service. As a result there may be a loss of monetary and "psychic income," which impacts directly upon one's mental health.

There is usually a direct relationship between earnings and social status. After retirement many individuals are compelled to accept a lower-paying and lower-status position than the one previously held in the uniformed services. Status mobility upward or downward may precipitate stress not only for the military retiree, but other family members as well. It is not uncommon for an upwardly mobile husband to "outgrow" his wife while she remains much as she was at the time of their marriage. Family members may also direct hostility toward what they perceive as the aggravating object, the retiree.

In a study of military family dynamics, Giffen and McNeil (1967) interviewed family members regarding their perceptions of the mental health impact of retirement on the family unit. Almost invariably when the retiree was asked how the family was affected by the retirement, the response was that they had not been affected. Without being asked, one wife volunteered, "It hurts me to see my husband start at the bottom again; I also hate to see other people get credit for what he does and that's what his present boss is doing." Still another wife related an incident in which a neighbor asked their ten year old son what he liked most about the military service and he responded that "I liked the fact that my father was an officer and I was somebody." A retiree's eighteen year old daughter remarked pitifully that her father was "smart enough to do more than he is doing now." Thus, the retiree and the retiree's family encounter potential stresses as retirement is faced and these stresses are related to the age of the retiree and the nature of the military social system itself.

The Military Social System

The military community is a relatively distinct social system that, prior to World War II, traditionally dictated its own patterns of behavior. As is true in other social systems, career military personnel and their families internalized the codes and values of this community, incorporating them as a way of life (Janowitz, 1960). Whereas significant changes have occurred within the present day military service, important aspects of the earlier days remain.

Within this social system, roles and statuses have been fairly clearly defined and accepted. Many of the role and status expectations have been codified into regulations and deviations from these standards are not accepted by other system members in a kindly manner. Because the career military person has spent the major portion of his/her adult life in this social system, movement to the civilian world may represent an unknown and a time of crisis that disrupts the retiree's equilibrium because previously used coping mechanisms are ineffective. Various writers have offered different theoretical perspectives to explain what happens to the retiree. McNeil and Giffen (1967) for example, utilize role theory; Milowe (1964) used Erickson's ego theory; Greenberg (1965) suggests depression as an explanation; Druss (1965) uses a combination of social and psychoanalytic theory; and Kilpatrick and Kilpatrick (1979) utilize grief theory; Doherty (1982) believes crisis theory is appropriate. Each of these perspectives will be briefly discussed, but the ideology suggested by crisis theory will be dealt with first because it is believed that each of the other explanatory perspectives have the potentiality to emerge at a time of crisis such as retirement from active duty.

Crisis Theory and Military Retirement

A crisis may be defined as "a period of disequilibrium, overpowering the individual's homeostatic mechanisms" (Parad and Caplan, 1960). Caplan offers a working definition stating that "a crisis occurs when a person faces an obstacle to important life goals that is, for a time, insurmountable through the utilization of his customary methods of problem-solving" (Caplan, 1961). A crisis has five components: an event that is perceived to be hazardous, the vulnerable state, the precipitating factor, the state of active crisis, and the stage of resolution or crisis resolution (Golan, 1978). A crisis may occur in anyone's life and may be triggered by any event that happens throughout a lifetime. In order for a crisis to occur, however, the event must be perceived as being hazardous. A crisis for one person is not necessarily a crisis for another person. In fact, an event may be seen differently by an individual at different points in time. The Chinese written character for crisis can be interpreted both as danger or opportunity (Golan, 1978). Among the numerous events that may trigger a crisis are such things as marriage, divorce, birth of a child, loss of a job, or loss of a love object.

Experiencing a crisis is not suggestive of psychopathology but rather a transitory occurrence, an episode that has overpowered the individual's usual coping mechanisms. Crisis theory presupposes a relatively stable individual who is reasonably absent of significant psychopathology. Retirement from the military service may been by some career personnel as a hazardous event, thereby disturbing their equilibrium. Military retirement probably creates some amount of anxiety and apprehension for each retiree and his/her family, though the level of disequilibrium is minimal for most. Milowe (1964), however, has observed that there is a statistically significant increase in the symptoms that are psychological in nature presented by those approaching retirement. Figure 4.1 illustrates the crisis course. It can be seen that retirement may be a crisis stimulus for the susceptible individual. Although the level of functioning may be disequilibrated for a period

Figure 4.1
Crisis Course for Susceptible Individual

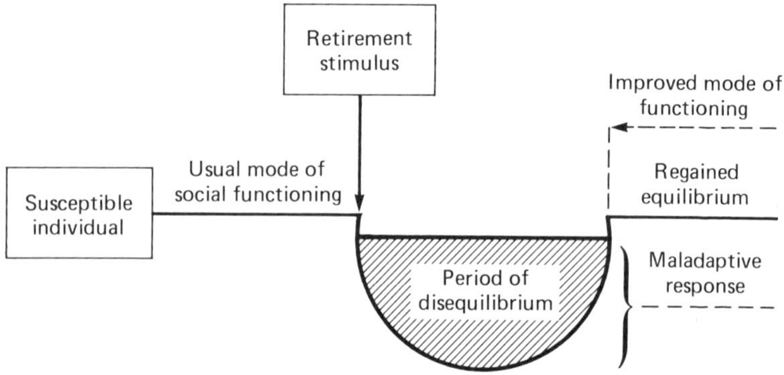

of time, there is a great likelihood the individual will emerge from the period of crisis functioning at the previous level or at an improved level of functioning (Giffen and McNeil, 1967).

Retirement can be a growth experience for the individual or it may lead to a maladaptive adjustment. Several theories have been offered to explain the susceptibility of some people to the event of retirement from the military service, but military retirement is perceived as a hazardous event often enough to be labeled the "retirement syndrome" (McNeil and Giffen, 1967).

The Retirement Syndrome: An Analysis

Milowe (1964) published the first article that focused upon the mental health aspects of military retirement. Milowe, however, directed his attention toward the preretirement phase of retirement. Although Milowe entitled his paper "A Study in Role Diffusion . . . ," which implies a use of role theory, in actuality he relies upon psychoanalytic theory and, more specifically, ego theory as explicated by Eric Erickson.

Erickson identifies eight stages that people transcend. Four of these stages occur during childhood: basic trust vs. mistrust, autonomy vs. shame and doubt, initiative vs. guilt, and industry vs. inferiority. It is necessary for the individual to negotiate successfully the stages of childhood before being prepared to tackle the tasks associated with adulthood. The adult tasks begin at adolescence with identity vs. role confusion, and in the progress to young adulthood, the task is intimacy vs. isolation. In adulthood the tasks are generativity vs. stagnation followed by ego integrity vs. despair as one reaches maturity (Erickson, 1963). Milowe further suggests that career service personnel who encounter mental health problems when confronted with retirement had "major crises early in life, predisposing toward a turbulent adolescence." Many neurotic trends were therefore unresolved making successful transition through the adolescent stage of identity vs. role confusion at best extremely difficult. Becoming a career member of the uniformed services offered them a solution because it provided an identity. Unfortunately this identity was only temporary, a "pseudomoratorium" that sufficed until they approached retirement. Previously unresolved mental health problems emerge thus rendering them unable to cope with the crisis of retirement. In addition, Milowe suggests the need for further scientific exploration of this phenomenon in order to develop preventive mental health strategies.

Druss (1965) views military retirement as a crisis point in the life of the career soldier in two separate but related areas. These areas may be considered external and internal. External factors include social, economic, and factual problems that could be, at least theoretically, handled on the level of practical advice and guidance. Internal problems are intrapsychic conflicts of a neurotic and unrealistic nature that require the skills of a trained mental health professional to treat adequately.

The main external social problem faced by most retirees is their need to maintain adequate income levels. Retirees recognize the need to work, but experience concern about the transferability of skills learned in the military service to the civilian labor market. In addition, a second major concern relates to the selection of a retirement residence. Career service personnel are, in a sense, migrants and as such are not likely to have close ties to any particular community or any place they can call "home." Consequently, many retirees are predisposed to settle near military installations in selecting a final residence.

Internal or intrapsychic problems revolve around three aspects of fear and loss: 1. fear of loss of power and authority, 2. fear of loss of a familiar way of life, and 3. fear of loss of security. By the time they attain retirement eligibility, career military personnel are likely to be in positions that afford them considerable power and authority. Loss of this position evokes fears of impending impotence and uselessness. Twenty or more years with the same institution develops a knowledge of the intricacies of the system that is available only to one who "learned the ropes." The prospective retiree thus faces an unknown and unfamiliar arena, the civilian environment. To many, the military service is viewed as the epitome of security and retirement represents a loss of this security. One or more of these fears may be experienced by the prospective retiree and at such a high level of stress that his/her equilibrium is seriously disturbed.

Druss (1965) believes that the retirement crisis can be minimized or avoided if adequate preventive health services were provided to the preretiree. He suggests that these services be made mandatory if necessary.

Greenberg (1965) analyzes military retirement within the context of depression and offers that it is a "depressive equivalent" that mirrors the description of the "Old Soldier Syndrome." The afflicted prospective retiree presents depressive symptoms with psychological as well as physical components. Greenberg develops his theory of depression out of psychoanalytic theory. It is suggested that retirement symbolizes rejection to the old soldier syndrome and unconsciously the retiree moves to reject the military establishment before it can reject him. Greenberg therefore focuses solely upon the preretirement phase of retirement, neglecting in his analysis problems associated with post-retirement. Depressive equivalents are not necessarily classic symptoms of depression but may be acted out behaviorally. Perhaps a major contribution made by Greenberg is his observation that the preretiree may engage in a single act of flagarantly unacceptable behavior that forces the attention of the military upon the prosective retiree. These flagrant acts are out of character for the individual and includes such incidents as being absent without leave (AWOL), committing homosexual acts, pedophilia, or crimes like theft. These self-destructive behaviors can be seen as depressive equivalent. Similar to other writers, Greenberg stresses the need for further research and the development of preventive mental health measures.

McNeil and Giffen (1967), in studying military retirement, coined the use of the concept "the retirement syndrome." They countered that "pre-retirement symptoms appear often enough and at times are severe enough to be classified as a classic syndrome. While the symptoms are not of themselves unique, the precipitating cause, early retirement, is." In an earlier publication, McNeil and Giffen (1965b) explain the retirement process in terms of a crisis. They point out the necessity of preretirement planning that should begin, at a minimum, at least one year before the anticipated retirement date. Planning must be done in four crucial areas: 1. retirement activity (usually this means employment), 2. retirement residence, 3. finances, and 4. appraisal of health. Appropriate planning in these areas would channel anxiety constructively and therefore decrease the likelihood of experiencing a crisis state at the time of retirement. Although McNeil and Giffen differentiate three phases of a retirement continuum—preretirement, a period of role confusion, and eventual adjustment or maladjustment—the heart of their role theory conceptualization is found in the second phase. Their analysis of role confusion as a concept is discussed below, and while the study was published in 1965, the findings appear pertinent today. If concepts like "double-dipping" were included in their perspective, or if federal civil service employment as well as defense industry jobs were included, comments made about military retirement today would be quite similar.

The period immediately following retirement from the armed forces is a most difficult time for the retiree. He is in the throes of adjusting from a military career to a civilian setting. This period can be called a time of role confusion. "Role" in this context refers to an individual's behavior in various situations. When roles are clearly defined we have a clear picture of expected behavior. The mere mention of the term is usually sufficient to trigger a mental image. For example, if we say "priest," most think of a religious and devout individual wearing ecclesiastical garments. When roles are clearly defined, both the particular individual performing the role and society have reached some type of agreement regarding the expected performance of the role player. To use the above example, when an individual visits a priest, each knows his role and performs accordingly.

Such a clear definition or understanding of roles is not always the case. Role expectations for some groups and/or individuals have not been clearly defined. If there is uncertainty of role performance both on the part of the individual (retiree) and society, this uncertainty produces role confusion or ambiguity. In role confusion we are assuming that the individual concerned is willing and able to perform the role but lacks sufficient knowledge to do so. Role confusion contrasts with role conflict; here the role performance is known but for some reason the individual does not perform the expected role. The retired military person usually wants to make an adjustment to civilian life but is hampered because his role has not been clearly defined.

Society has failed to define or structure a realistic role for the retired military person, who is usually visualized as either occupying a lucrative position in a large corporation that does volume business with the Department of Defense or as living a life of leisure on a comfortable pension. To society the retired military person's role is placed at extreme ends of a continuum, where the majority do not fall, and overlooks the space between these poles where the greatest percentage of retirees are to be found.

There is a marked contrast in roles between a military and a nonmilitary setting, between active duty and retired status. This is dramatized when one reflects briefly upon the military structure itself. There is a built-in status structure within the military establishment. Each individual's role is predetermined through tradition and written regulation. The uniform and its accompanying insignia determines the role of the individual in relation to all others within the military society. Deviation from expected role performance is dealt with swiftly and at times harshly. Upon retirement this symbolization and structuring of roles is lost. It is also extremely unlikely that the retired individual will make a lateral transfer in a new career to a status equal to that previously held. Generally, the retiree must start at the bottom of the ladder, which represents a considerable loss of financial and psychic income.

There are several reasons why the retiree usually must start at the bottom. Among these is the fact that most industries tend to promote from within their own ranks. A new employee generally must prove his/her value to the company to move successively through increasingly responsible positions. Another factor is the extent of transferability of skills. Skills used in the military service are not always immediately transferable to civilian occupations. For example, an aircraft commander on a bomber may be far advanced on the administrative ladder of operations officer. Administrative skills are considered to be easily transferred. While an operations officer's function is managerial and administrative in nature, it is still geared to combat. It is quite possible that these skills may be exceedingly difficult if not virtually impossible to transfer. Another important factor is the extent of civilian prejudice against military retirees. It is often believed the military retiree relies upon authority and force rather than arbitration and negotiation to resolve conflict. This prejudice may be displayed through the tendency of civilian employers to underpay the labor of the retiree, who must often assume a lower-status position with consequently less authority and responsibility. The retiree may find that considerable emphasis is placed upon individual achievement whereas in the military service there tends to be greater reliance upon teamwork and group effort.

The military retiree is at a further disadvantage because he/she has not been accustomed to bargaining for wages since the armed forces salary scales are legislated by Congress and everyone of similar rank and seniority receive equal pay.

Many retirees enter the civilian labor market with expectations of a salary commensurate with that which they received while on active duty. This, in fact, seldom occurs. It is a disturbing experience for the retirees to learn that their worth to the potential employer is valued so lowly. Where the individual expected to have a greatly increased income upon retirement, retired pay and earnings from the civilian employment combined may be less than active duty pay. This is especially true for the serviceperson who has received incentive or hazardous duty pay in addition to base pay and allowances. In our culture, type of employment and earnings are indices of social position. The loss of "psychic income" becomes concretized through actual loss in earning power.

The retired military person may be the focus of opposition originating from fellow employees. The retiree may be seen as an outsider who has not "grown up" with the company; yet, he/she either occupies a promotional position or is in active competition for it. In a supervisory position, the retiree must be very careful not to "pull rank" in order to avoid being caricatured as a maladjusted "old soldier." Resentment may also be present if it is thought the retiree, by holding a position, is preventing a civilian from being employed who has no additional source of income. Fellow employees may also be envious of the fact that the retiree receives retirement pay in addition to earnings from the current employment.

Members of the retiree's family also experience role confusion. A wife assumes the status level of her husband and shares his position in the social system. The military wife who has become accustomed to expect special treatment because of her husband's rank experiences some moments of alarm and dismay when these are no longer accorded. Children also experience a phase of readjustment and, in many instances, need to search for a new identity.

Role confusion, thus, is an inescapable experience for all military retirees. The period of role confusion may have a decided effect upon the individual's eventual adjustment to retirement.

Doherty examined the crisis theory approach in greater depth in an unpublished Ph.D. dissertation (1982). He suggested that the idea of crisis could not be accepted in isolation but must include concepts of adaptation, coping processes, object relations, and the system entry factor of adolescent identity formation.

In studying adaptation, Doherty focused upon the mid-life task areas of household management, parenting, and career management. He sought information about role performance in various social positions and how the individual feels about role performance and role change. Coping processes included three psychological factors—recognition, mastery, and resolution. Object relations added the dimension of personality to the retirement adjustment process. The system of adolescent identity formation is borrowed from Erickson (1963) as explicated by Milowe (1964) and his theory of pseudomoratorium. Doherty believes the level of identity formation achieved by the individual at the time of entry into the military service will be predictive of the difficulty experienced at the time of retirement. Doherty, therefore, expands the concept of crisis to include other psychological variables that seem to impact upon both the preretirement and post-retirement process.

Kilpatrick and Kilpatrick published a review article in 1979 dealing with the mental health problems of military retirees. After reviewing the relatively few studies published during the past several years and drawing upon their own clinical experience, they concluded that the crisis of military retirement should be studied within the construct of mourning reactions. According to the authors, mourning is preceded by a loss or perceived threat of a loss and retirement from the military service represents a loss for the career service person. The loss, however, may be attached to any love object (e.g., a loved one, prestige or status, health, a job, or a prized possession).

When one suffers a loss and mourns, a predictable cycle of grief inevitably must occur. Following the recognition of the loss, the individual protests the loss and makes an effort to recover the lost object. At this time there may be depressive symptoms such as crying, pain, loss of appetite, sleep disturbance and/or physical problems. Despair follows the protest stage and the existent depressive symptoms may become more severe and impinge upon the social functioning of the mourner. Next follows a period of detachment, which is marked by decreased socialization, absent spontaniety, and bland expression. The final phase of the mourning process occurs when the individual begins to recover. The lost object is placed in its proper perspective with the passage of time.

Kilpatrick and Kilpatrick also suggest that invariably all military retirees go through this grief process, although all retirees may not experience an acute grief reaction. They stress further the need for preretirement preparatory programs and professional intervention for individuals who are more severely affected.

Each of the authors highlighted above discuss the need for a systematic retirement preparatory program. They acknowledge generally that relatively few persons experience severe incapacitating problems relating to retirement but recognize the potential susceptibility of any retiree. In view of this, preventive programs are strongly encouraged. These programs should focus on the retirement continuum as well as benefits available to the retiree and his/her family. Retirement preparatory programs, however, raise the issue of the extent of employer responsibility in the area of employee retirement adjustment. There are varied opinions that range from practically no responsibility to those who believe the employer has considerable responsibility. The individual retiree also has responsibility, and a satisfactory balance between employer and employee activity impacts upon the mental health parameters of the retiree and his/her family.

Retirement and Employer Responsibility

Private industry, as well as the military service, have never really resolved satisfactorily the question regarding the extent of employer responsibility toward the prospective retiree, the retired person, or their families. Opinions vary from those who believe the employer has no responsibility to those who argue the employer should assure to every extent possible the maximum adjustment in retirement. Since the passage of the Social Security Act, most employers have come to accept the right of employees to pension benefits. In spite of this trend, thousands of industrial employees have learned at the point of retirement that their expected pension is not available. Federal legislation has been enacted to minimize the possibility of this tragedy. If employers were placed on a continuum, their position relative to retirement could be located anywhere between the two poles (i.e., complete responsibility to no responsibility).

The military service has been legally committed to a pension responsibility since 1861. During the preretirement phase, the military service seemingly has never been fully committed to an individualized preparatory assistance approach. Individuals approaching retirement are briefed and provided reading materials. Limited job referral resources have been provided utilizing the existing state employment agencies. At one time assistance was available in many places for things such as resume preparation. For example, Program Transition was one individualized effort. In this program, active duty personnel were released from normal military duty functions in order that they could learn a skill that could be sold in the civilian labor market. Program Transition was designed primarily for young persons completing their military obligation who did not have marketable skills to sell in the civilian labor market. The program was extended to include prospective career military retirees. Budgetary retrenchment, however, forced the discontinuance of Program Transition and most other individualized programs in the retirement preparatory phase.

During the post-retirement period, the military service has fluctuated along the employer responsibility continuum. A case in point is the provision of medical care for retirees and their dependents. Medical services have always been provided to dependents and retired personnel on a space-available basis. This worked quite well when the number of persons on the retired rolls was relatively small. Now, at many military installations, medical care for retirees and their families is practically nonexistent. Although retirees and their dependents are included under the coverage of the military medicare program (CHAMPUS), the retiree's co-insurance share is larger than that for dependents of active duty personnel and benefits are fewer, especially those benefits relating to handicapped children.

Another crucial post-retirement benefit is the eligibility of surviving dependents to receive cash payments derived from the deceased retiree's pension rights. Such a program is in effect in the military services through the Family Protection Plan. This was developed as an actuarially sound survivorship annuity. If the retiree participates in the plan, each month an actuarially determined percentage of his retired pay is deducted to pay for the annuity selected. Annuities are available in the amounts of one-eighth, one-fourth, or one-half of the retiree's retirement pay. The plan has been criticized as being too expensive and too restrictive (U.S. Congress, Subcommittee on Survivor Benefits, 1980). A small percentage of eligible retirees elect to utilize this form of insurance protection for their families. For the maximum annuity of one-half of retired pay, depending upon the ages of the retiree and the spouse, the cost of the family protection can be as much as one-fourth of the monthly retired pay check. Recently, however, some of the more objectionable features have been literalized (Hearings, *Benefits for Survivors of Retired Military Personnel,* 1980).

Within the past twenty years, the overall direction of the military service on the employer responsibility continuum has been toward less responsibility. Experience has shown that many retirees desire and need more assistance than has been made available to them. There is greater need for help in the areas of resume preparation, job placement, vocational guidance and counseling, financial planning, and counseling to assist in dealing with the "psychological shock." Adequate assistance programs should begin many months or even a few years prior to actual retirement and continue afterwards where needed. Theoretically, the best retirement planning begins the day the career military person enters on active duty. One beneficial program no longer in operation was the policy of allowing individuals approaching retirement to select the geographic area of choice for their final duty assignment. This gave the family a "head start" on retirement. Obviously many things could be done to assist the retiree, but such programs are low-priority items.

The mental health of the retiree and his/her family is inextricably tied to the peace of mind of the individuals involved. Peace of mind suggests that some level of satisfaction has been achieved. As will be shown below, adequate retirement preparation and subsequent satisfactory adjustment requires activity in several areas.

Parameters for Good Mental Health in Retirement

The period preceding retirement can be a most difficult time for the military person as well as for the family. The career military person may begin to think about the "good old days" and become nostalgic or may begin to wonder about the future and experience a rise in anxiety. Most individuals do not experience stress of a sufficiently severe degree to have their equilibrium overpowered; however, the likelihood of this can be reduced significantly if there is adequate preparation for retirement.

Individuals approaching retirement may respond to this eventually in individualized fashions, but essentially it tends toward active or passive preparation. The extent of planning may be evaluated relative to how effectively the prospective retiree has been prepared in four important areas. These areas are: 1. retirement activity, 2. retirement residence, 3. finances, and 4. appraisal of health. For most retired military personnel the primary retirement activity will be employment. This entails a careful evaluation of individual skills and interests and how these may be utilized in nonmilitary occupational pursuits. Active planning necessitates some realistic decision regarding the geographic area in which it is desired to pursue one's retirement activity. Some financial reserve is important so that one is not pressured into making premature decisions regarding retirement activity or residence. When there is urgent need for additional funds, it becomes quite difficult to make decisions selectively and wisely. Nowadays the condition of health need not be a major factor except for those individuals who are retired because of medical disability.

A person who has actively prepared for retirement will have asked and effectively answered these three questions:

1. What do I want to do?
2. Where do I want to do it?
3. Is it feasible for me to do what I want, where I want to do it?

For most career personnel, retirement from the military service presents an unknown. Approaching an unfamiliar situation can be an anxiety-producing experience. Constructive channeling of this will, in all probability, propel the prospective retiree toward actively preparing for retirement. Lack of this will impede effective pre-retirement preparatory activity (McNeil and Giffen, 1965a).

Making a satisfactory adjustment to retirement requires conscious activity on the part of the retiree. The term "adjustment" appears to be relatively easy to understand until one begins examining its components. We are generally hard-pressed to justify why it is thought that a specific individual is adjusted or maladjusted. We are also frequently inclined to think of adjustment merely as personal happiness and contentment. In our culture, it appears that adjustment implies much more than this. There are at least three specific aspects to adjustment: 1. personal happiness, 2. meeting expectations, and 3. exhibiting some evidence of achievement. These components doubtlessly overlap, but each retains a degree of independence. For example, to be personally happy one usually must meet societal expectations. On the other hand, an individual can be exhibiting some evidence of achievement yet not be happy.

Without a doubt, most retirees make a good adjustment to civilian life. The quality of this adjustment, however, is difficult to evaluate. It is doubtful that one can completely give up an experience that has patterned the greater portion of an adult life without some observable signs or symptoms. To measure the adjustment is, at best, difficult. Some insight into the extent of the adjustment can be gained if some consideration is given the following factors: 1. job satisfaction, 2. satisfaction with retirement residence, 3. maintenance of an accustomed standard of living, and 4. happiness of the family with retirement.

Job satisfaction implies success in changing from a military career to a civilian career. Work itself is an important ingredient in the life of every adult male, and a retiree who is not engaged in constructive employment will experience a certain degree of maladjustment. Unhappiness with one's retirement residence may tend to magnify other dissatisfactions and invariably cause some degree of maladjustment.

Some retired personnel attempt to circumvent or lessen the trauma of retirement by retaining as much of the military symbolism as possible. This may be accomplished by developing and cementing friendships with personnel still on active duty or by seeking social relationships with individuals who are similarly retired. It is probably not accidental that retired military personnel tend to cluster in certain geographic areas. About 17 percent settle in California, 10 percent in Florida, and 10 percent in Texas. This may reflect a conscious or unconscious desire to avoid the pain of role confusion associated with life in a nonmilitary environment and may serve to bolster the ego of the retiree and reduce the anxiety that occurs with loss of identity. The success of the Retired Officers Association is, in part, attributable to the fact that they all are in the same boat.

Maintenance of an accustomed standard of living has far-reaching implications for the retiree and his family. If the retired individual finds it necessary to radically reduce his standard of living, this is ego-deflating. It may imply to him and others inadequacy or inability to compete successfully in the civilian labor market. Failure to compete would probably suggest that the individual is a misfit who can only function in the military setting. This may well act as a focal point for maladjustive behaviors and accompanying increases in psychological symptoms and lessened individual productivity. Along with this, familial happiness is also an important concern. It can be assumed that family members, unhappy with retirement, will create or intensify the difficulty for the retiree (McNeil and Giffen, 1965a).

Recommendations

Approximately 40,000 individuals retire from the military each year. The potential within this group of new retirees is impressive. Unfortunately, many undergo stresses that are sometimes quite damaging to their concept of self, but fortunately there are health and social services available to minimize the difficulties associated with military retirement. The following recommendations represent a growing sensitivity to problems of military retirees and merit serious consideration by policy makers, the military community, career military personnel and their families, and helping professionals:

1. Establish good communication between the career military person and his/her family so that mutual support and planning is possible.
2. Educate civilian health practitioners on the etiology and symptomology of the retirement syndrome. It would appear that successful work with a military retiree (and his/her family members) would require extensive knowledge of military life.

3. Provide routine assistance to military persons in developing a realistic preretirement plan. Such a program would channel anxiety and energy in a constructive fashion as well as initiating other careers early in the planning process (McNeil and Giffen, 1965a). Ogburn, et al., (1969) suggests that such planning begin when one decides on a career in the military. Certainly, planning should begin several years before retirement.
4. Provide low-level supportive counseling to all individuals nearing retirement age to assist in minimizing their confusion and anxiety, and enhancing their functioning.
5. Provide spouses and children supportive services as they prepare for changes associated with the family member's retirement and need to develop coping strategies.
6. Allow the military Mental Hygiene Consultation Services staff access to economic, educational, and vocational information so that assistance in these areas could be provided (Druss, 1965).
7. Provide training programs during the earlier years of the individual's career. Such training might include information on self-awareness and self-acceptance. It might assist the individual to look backward at accomplishments, assess himself, and look forward to his future life (Bradford, 1979). One successful program is called PREP (Pre-Retirement Education Program). The program prepares the individual for the future. It is a dynamic, provocative, informative, and enjoyable group experience. The program discusses topics on adjustment, well-being, health, legal affairs, income planning, and peace of mind (West, 1980).
8. Provide opportunities for military persons to increase those skills that would facilitate entry into civilian life.
9. Provide an orientation to civilian life that focuses on such things as new demands, different expectations, and civilian views of the military.
10. Develop groups for military retirees to provide support as the transition from military to civilian life is encountered.

11. Spot individuals who may be high emotional risks early and assist them in the transition from military life.
12. Encourage the retiree to develop multiple skills. Variety is a lifesaver when the regular skill does not provide employment.
13. Assist individuals in working through grief associated with the loss involved in retirement (Kilpatrick and Kilpatrick, 1979).

5

PROBLEMS, PROSPECTS, AND TRENDS

The purpose of this book has been to examine within a historical framework the economic, social, and psychological dilemmas of military retirement. In explicating the various themes of the book, we have focused our attention on the impact of retirement on the retiree, his family, and society. The retirement of military personnel from active duty does not fit the classical model of occupational retirement and as a result, it does not conform to what most people have in mind when they think of retirement (e.g., that a person significantly reduces or does not continue his/her participation in the labor market and goes on to lead a life of contentment and leisure). To the contrary, military retirement, in the conventional sense, has meant that a vast majority of those who have retired from active duty have not completely removed themselves from participation in the civilian labor market. The benefits that accrue to retirees through the current military pension system, for the most part, are inadequate to support them and their families and forces them to seek post-retirement employment. Work beyond retirement serves both as a source of financial gain and psychological reward for the individual and his/her family.

The pronounced trend toward larger and larger numbers of retirees, the natures of the environment in which retirement takes place, continual economic stagnation and rapid inflation and the nature of the retirement experience itself establish parameters for discussing policies and alternative policies related to the current system. Economic policies, problems, and trends emerge as issues of primary importance.

Primary Trends in Military Retirement

Three primary trends seem to have charted the course that led to the current economic issues so prominent today in the military retirement program. These trends are: 1. humanitarianism, 2. personal management strategies, and 3. control.

The humanitarian motive provided the most persistent impetus for the initiation and perpetuation of the military retirement system. This is demonstrated vividly in the disability retirement program. Although disability benefits may have served a recruitment purpose, it was essentially the way the public had of assuming financial responsibility for the service person and his/her dependents. Programs initiated during times of war tend to be humanitarian to the extent long-term policy implications and future costs may not get the careful, studied attention they deserve. The nondisability retirement program legislated during the Civil War attempted to blend humanitarian and personnel management strategies into a viable piece of legislation. This statute did indeed meet an immediate and long-term need, but again future costs were not projected adequately.

As the size of the retired rolls grew, an attempt was made to control their size by limiting the number of persons who could be on the retired rolls at any given time. Subsequently control was embodied in the legislation to limit the earnings of retired personnel and/or restrict their retirement options. Control and humanitarianism influenced personnel management strategies, sometimes as allies, but also at times as antagonists. No satisfactory method was found, or perhaps seriously sought, to bring these three themes together. As indicated earlier, no actuarial study was made of the cost of the military retirement program for almost one hundred years after it started. So today there is monumental concern about the unfunded liability. In a similar vein military personnel were included in the social security program as a humanitarian effort without studying fully its implications. Presently an action to control costs by integration of retired pay with social security benefits will cause the retiree to receive less money than if he/she had never been covered under social security.

As concern increases regarding the cost of military retirement, humanitarianism has been pushed to a less prominent position while personnel management and control have moved to the forefront. The personnel management quandary probably will not be resolved until policy planners come to grips with the youth and vigor concept. Control, therefore becomes a primary mechanism or tactic to solve the economic problems of retirement. Control and its essential ingredient, power, can easily be used in a negative or coercive manner. Many military personnel, both active duty and retired, believe that control is already being used coercively. The term "double dipper" is reflective of this attitude. When President Carter used the term to characterize military retirees, it was given a quality of legitimacy thereby encouraging everyone to view the military retiree in a negative light. Attitudes such as these lead to covert or overt hostility toward the retiree and ultimately to more controlling legislation.

Illustrative of this trend is the tenor of published material in the past few years regarding military retirement, most of which is negative (Binkin and Kryiakopoulos, 1981; R.V.L. Cooper, 1981; Reed, 1975). A danger of this type of mentality is that controlling measures may neglect to evaluate future implications and compound the problems that developed through an essentially humanitarian philosophy. The negativism creates a societal paradox for the retiree. Retirement from the military service may have been mandatory or strongly encouraged by military retirement policies, yet society greets the retiree with antagonism. Retirement to leisure at an early age is frowned upon and earning a salary while drawing retired pay brings forth the label of "double dipper." Control therefore, which may be coercive, is seen at the governmental level as well as the peer level. Although economic reform appears to be needed, the primary impetus should not come from the control ideology. Control acts as a backlash to humanitarian activities instead of being an integral part of short- and long-term planning, and impacts directly upon policies that relate to the effects of inflation.

The Effects of Inflation

The effects of inflation upon the real value of retirees' pension benefits is a central policy issue in the development of services for this group. Inflation has two distinct effects upon pension benefits accruing to retirees: one is the day-to-day erosion of their accustomed standards of living; the second is the uncertainty about the future real value of their benefits (Morse and Gray, 1980). It seems desirable that future retirement policies attempt to minimize the manifest as well as latent effects of inflation on pension benefits. One plausible alternative to countering the effects of inflation upon benefits is to implement a program whereby active duty careerists would be able to make voluntary contributions to increase their post-retirement incomes. Since career service personnel differ in their needs for income before and after retirement, they should have options for contributing differential amounts. By building up a greater equity in their pensions, retirees will have a partial hedge against erosion from inflation.

The erosion of the real value of pension benefits caused by inflation combined with high unemployment and limited job availability in the civilian labor sector may also have significant effects upon the frequency with which career service personnel retire and the length of time they choose to remain on active duty. Because of the instability in the economy, careerists eligible for retirement after having served twenty years may not be willing to elect the voluntary retirement option. This will be particularly the case for individuals who are systematically promoted and who are not forced to retire upon completion of a specified career length (thirty years or less, dependent upon the grade attained before promotion failure). Thus, at a minimum, the continuance of high-level inflation and high unemployment in the labor market are likely to be important factors leading some to extend their date of retirement. Economic issues are inextricably intertwined with social issues; in fact, at times it is impossible to separate one from the other. Second-career options, prospects, and pursuits demonstrate this inseparability.

Retirees and Second Careers

Retirement from the armed services generally occurs between forty and fifty years of age, when most individuals are relatively healthy and productive (Platte, 1976). For the majority of those who retire, complete or full retirement at this age is not feasible. Movement into second careers in the civilian labor market has become the preferred pattern over the years. Retirees in this transitional stage, however, must find new job opportunities, get retraining if necessary, finance, in part, moving expenses if this is required, and maintain their emotional equilibrium as well as that of their families during the period between jobs (Dumas, 1977). The burden of meeting these responsibilities can be greatly enhanced by the availability of appropriate second-career assistance programs. Hence, in a broad policy sense, it is not too difficult to formulate reasonable alternatives for assisting retirees seeking civilian careers. One such alternative, we posit, is a system-wide, coordinated program of employment services designed to specifically make retirees (both pre- and post-retirees) aware of the nature and location of new employment opportunities that best match their skills. In conjunction with an early preretirement counseling program, these will be immensely important in enabling retirees (and their families) to plan effectively for future contingencies.

Another alternative would be the development of a program in which the federal government could provide special tax or other incentives for employers to sign conditional employment contracts with retirees during the transition period that, in effect, guarantee the retiree a job upon successful completion of a program of retraining (Dumas, 1977). In this way retirees requiring minimal or extensive retraining would have some assurance that undertaking training in a particular area of civilian employment would provide them with a relatively rewarding and attractive job. Furthermore, during the period of transition from military to civilian life, there appears to be a need for a policy and program that systematically provides immediate monetary benefits to offset the adverse financial maladies associated with having to begin a second career in mid-life. Without a specific retirement policy that assures some financial assistance during the transition period, the military system may find it exceedingly difficult to retain the kinds of career personnel it needs most (R.V.L. Cooper, 1981).

The Extent of the Military's Responsibility

Neither private industry nor the military service have ever really resolved satisfactorily the question regarding the extent of employer responsibility toward prospective retirees, retired persons, or their families. Opinions vary from those who believe the employer has no responsibility to those who argue the employer should assure to every extent possible maximum adjustment in retirement, which in the military service includes establishing a second career. Individual retirees and their families do have a responsibility to prepare themselves for retirement, and most career service persons probably do make some plans for retirement, but the thoroughness of these plans may leave much to be desired.

We strongly contend that it is the military system that has the ultimate responsibility of making the transition from the military to civilian life a less traumatic process and one that is optimistic and realistic. This responsibility overlaps with the military's commitment to the total family. Unfortunately the military service has no organized program to provide assistance to individuals and their families who are making the transition. Several writers have pointed out the need for such services

(McNeil, 1964; Druss, 1965; Doherty, 1982). Doherty (1982), for example, makes some cogent, persuasive arguments for transitional services. He suggests that those who enter the military are systematically deprogrammed from a civilian culture and reprogrammed to the culture and values of the military world. Throughout the individual's military tenure these values are systematically reinforced and no effort is made at the end of the military career to reprogram the individual back to a civilian *modus operandi.*

Moreover, Doherty also suggests other reasons that transitional services could prove beneficial to the military establishment. Individual careerists approaching retirement may experience fear and anxiety, thereby reducing their effectiveness and efficiency in performing their assigned military responsibilities. Preretirement preparatory programs might minimize or alleviate potential productivity losses among these personnel. For those in the post-military retirement phase, some assistance with mental health and social problems is available through civilian counseling programs. Programs operated by the military such as CHAMPUS (Civilian Health and Medical Program of the Uniform Services) are designed to ease the burden of transition from one environment to another; however, the continually rising costs of CHAMPUS have brought about structural and fiscal changes that in most cases have not been beneficial for the retiree and his/her family. For example, in 1975, program funding was removed from military departments and placed under the direct supervision of the Office of the Secretary of Defense. This change resulted in more than 99 percent drop in the CHAMPUS portion of the Medical Department operating budget for Fiscal Year 1975 down to $4 million, compared to $507.7 million for Fiscal Year 1974 (Annual Report, Army Surgeon General, 1975).

The continuation of such drastic cuts will have severe negative implications for active duty and retiree populations. During the mid-1970s, for example, the number of Army psychiatrists assigned worldwide declined to approximately 185. At this availability level, the provision of essential mental health services for active duty personnel was still possible, but the capability for meeting the mental health needs of retirees and their dependents continued to decline (Annual Report, Army Surgeon General, 1974). Increasingly, nonactive duty personnel were referred to civilian therapists under CHAMPUS. At the same time, however, under the pressure of severe budgetary problems, CHAMPUS was narrowing the range of services for which it would pay. The net result was a continuing squeeze on mental health services for dependents and retired personnel. Moreover, the likelihood of increasing the number of mental health professionals remains bleak as the demand for these services continues to escalate.

As pointed out in preceeding chapters, over 40,000 military personnel are retiring each year with a significant number needing some type of preparatory retirement and post-retirement adjustment services. Not to admit that military retirees are different from the traditional, sixty-five year old retiree is to bury one's head in the sand. The military retiree is different, retiring at the average age of forty and having special mental health problems associated with early retirement (i.e., issues relating to employment, family responsibility, lack of understanding of the competitive job market, special status, family network dynamics, and integration into a geographic area). As Janowitz (1960) points out, the retiree did not have the same kinds of problems to contend with while on active duty since the military interceded for him/her, so that military personnel and their families internalized the codes and values of this community and incorporated them as a way of life. Many of the needed services were provided to the military person thereby reducing his/her need to seek such things in the civilian community. Moreover, the retiree understood the process to attain these services, which were clearly defined and structured, whereas these same services in the civilian community are redefined, less structured, and are layered into a multitude of subsystems.

The changes immediately following retirement in employment and environment have important implications for the emotional equilibrium of retirees and their families. The anxieties and pressures experienced by many retirees in adjusting to new externalities are inevitably transferred onto their families. As a result, retirees and their families oftentimes experience the retirement syndrome (McNeil and Giffen, 1967). This, without a doubt, is a period in time when there is an acute need by many retirees and their families to have access to social services that are designed to prevent family disintegration and ease the transition from military to nonmilitary life.

What appears to be needed are systematic policies that will enable those retirees and their families experiencing maladjustment problems to get the needed help outside of the conventional military-sponsored programs such as CHAMPUS. One approach is the development of third-party subsidy programs to civilian social service agencies that can provide the services retirees and their families need during the transitional period. Costs for such programs could be controlled by 1. limiting the amount of the subsidy for retirees and their families to a specified maximum per year, and 2. establishing a time limit for receiving subsidized services after retirement (e.g., a maximum eligibility period of two years after official detachment from active duty).

The Impact of Military Retirement

One of the major propositions of this book is that large-scale retirement of career military personnel may create profound dilemmas for retirees, their families, communities in which they settle, and society as a whole. The few studies dealing with the sociological impacts of military retirement appear to substantiate, in part, this thesis (Biderman, 1959; 1964; 1971; 1973; McNeil and Giffen, 1965a; 1965b; 1967; Giffen and McNeil, 1967; Platte, 1976). Life changes such as military retirement are familial stresses that may have significant impacts upon the individual members of the family and the broader social order. How the family and social systems adapt or adjust to these stresses has been a subject of great concern to the military establishment but has received little systematic attention in the research literature (McCubbin, et al., 1976).

Research on military retirement, its influence upon retirees and their families, and its impact upon society has been, for the most part, sporadic, ill-conceived, and limited to clinical observation and descriptive survey reports. As a result, most of the existing studies in this area are subject to the same methodological criticism. First, few studies are available that have purposely set out to test specific research hypotheses. Rather what we have are studies that have started and ended as clinical or exploratory investigations with untested common-sense assumptions. Second, most of the studies that exist have employed nonprobability samples from available populations rather than employing samples that were randomly selected and representative of the entire retiree universe. Hence, the conclusions drawn from these studies have limited applicability and generalizability. Third, many of the existing studies are ex post facto in nature and have had to depend upon data collected retrospectively (McCubbin, et al., 1976). Finally, many of the available studies did not employ rigorous research designs and have tended to rely upon unsophisticated and simplistic statistical procedures (i.e., frequency and percentage distributions, and cross-tabulations), which lend themselves to misinterpretation through spurious relationships. Thus, the current body of research reveals little about the complex and dynamic interactional processes associated with military retirement. This body of research does not enhance our understanding of the causal relationships between factors and variables correlated with the retirement process.

Without a doubt, the process of retirement has a profound impact upon the retiree, his family and kin, and society, but to what degree this hypothesis is true and under what conditions remains to be empirically investigated. It is important to recognize that available studies, because of their limitations, are not in themselves sufficient to form a basis for prescribing specific policy changes that will address all of the immediate concerns of retirees and their families.

The history of the military retirement system is one of relative success. From its inception in 1861, it has grown enormously to occupy a pre-eminent position among military programs. The survival of military retirement as a permanent American institution is no longer an important political question; the relevant issues today concern the optimal marginal improvements in the program that will make it more effective and responsive in the future.

REFERENCES

Annual Report. FY 1974. The Surgeon General, U.S. Army. Department of the Army, Washington, D.C.

Annual Report. FY 1975. The Surgeon General, U.S. Army. Department of the Army, Washington, D.C.

Ayers, G. W. 1977. The military establishment and social welfare, past, present, and future? *Journal of Sociology and Social Welfare* 4:522-29.

Bankers Trust Company. 1975. *Study of Corporate Pension Plans.* New York.

Bernard, J. 1957. *Social Problems at Mid-Century.* New York: Dryden Press.

Biderman, A. 1959. The prospective impact of large-scale military retirement. *Social Problems* 71:84-90.

———. 1964. Sequels to a military career: The retired military professional. In M. Janowitz (ed.) *The New Military: Changing Patterns of Organization.* New York: Russell Sage Foundation, pp. 287-366.

———. 1974. The retired military. In R. Little (ed.), *Handbook of Military Institutions.* Beverly Hills, Calif.: Sage Publications, pp. 126-63.

———. 1973. Where do they go from here? Retired military in America. *The Annals of the American Academy of Political and Social Science,* pp. 147-61.

Biderman, A. and Sharp, L. M. 1968. The convergence of military and civilian occupational structures: Evidence from studies of military retired employment. *American Journal of Sociology,* 73:381-99.

Binkin, M. and Kryiakopoulos, I. 1981. *Paying The Modern Military.* Washington, D.C.: The Brookings Institution.

Bradford, L. 1979. Can you survive your retirement? *Harvard Business Review.*

Caplan, G. 1961. *An Approach to Community Mental Health.* New York: Grune and Stratton.

Church, A. T., III. 1979. *Retirement Accounting and the Unfunded Liability.* M. A. Thesis. Naval Postgraduate School, Monterey, Calif.

Committee on Veterans' Affairs. 1955. U.S. Congress, House of Representatives. *The Provision of Federal Benefits for Veterans.* Washington, D. C.: U. S. Gov't. Printing Office.

Cooper, B. 1970. *Inquiry Into Survivor Benefits.* U. S. House of Representatives, Armed Services Committee. Ninety-first Congress, Second Session.

Cooper, R. V. L. 1981 *Military Retirees' Post Service Earnings and Employment.* Santa Monica, Calif.: Rand Corporation.

Defense Manpower Commission. 1976. *Defense Manpower Commission Staff Studies and Supporting Papers.* Washington, D. C.: U. S. Gov't. Printing Office.

Defense Manpower Data Center. 1980. *Fiscal Year 1980 Statistical Report on Military Retirement.* Washington, D. C.: U. S. Gov't. Printing Office.

________ . 1981a. *Fiscal Year 1981 Statistical Report on Military Retirement.* Washington, D. C.: U. S. Gov't. Printing Office.

________ . 1981b. *Valuation of The Military Retirement System.* Washington, D. C.: U. S. Gov't Printing Office.

Devine, E. J. and Kuzmack, R. A. 1976. Integration of military retired pay and social security benefits: The attribution problem and its implications for the private sector. In *Defense Manpower Commission Staff Studies and Supporting Papers, Volume V, Compensation and Retirement.* Washington, D. C.: U. S. Gov't. Printing Office.

Doherty, Thomas F. 1982. *Patterns of Adaptation to Military Retirement: An Exploratory Study,* unpublished dissertation, Smith College.

Druss, R. G. 1965. Problems associated with retirement from the military. *Military Medicine* 130:4, 382-85.

Dumas, L. J. 1977. Conversation, productive efficiency and social welfare. *Journal of Sociology and Social Welfare* 4:567-96.

Erickson, E. H. 1963. *Childhood and Society.* 2nd edition. New York: W. W. Norton.

First Quadrennial Review of Military Compensation. 1969. Department of Defense. *Modernizing Military Pay.* Washington, D. C.: U. S. Gov't. Printing Office.

Frances, A. and Gale, L. 1973. Family structure and treatment in the military. *Family Process* 12:171-78.

Ganoe, W. A. 1942. *The History of the United States Army.* 2nd edition, revised. New York: Appleton-Century Co.

Giffen, M. B. and McNeil, J. S. 1967. Effect of military retirement on dependents. *Archives of General Psychiatry* 17:717-22.

Golan, N. 1978. *Treatment in Crisis Situations.* New York: Free Press.

Greenberg, H. R. 1965. Depressive equivalents in the pre-retirement years: The old soldier syndrome. *Military Medicine* 130:4, 251-55.

Hale, R. F. 1978. *The Military Retirement System: Options for Change.* Congressional Budget Office. Washington, D. C.: U. S. Gov't. Printing Office.

Hearings, *Employment of Retired Military and Civilian Personnel by Defense Industries.* 1959. Subcommittee of the House Armed Services Committee. Eighty-sixth Congress, First Session.

Hearings, *Report of The Special Subcommittee on Survivor Benefits of The Committee on Armed Services.* 1970. U. S. House of Representatives. Ninety-first Congress, Second Session.

Hearings, *The Disability Retirement of Gen. Earl E. Anderson.* 1975. U. S. Congress, House Subcommittee on Military Compensation on Armed Services. Ninety-Fourth Congress, First Session. No. 94-231.

Hearings, *Benefits for Survivors of Retired Military Personnel.* 1980. U. S. Congress, Military Compensation Subcommittee of The House Armed Services Committee. Ninety-sixth Congress, Second Session.

Hearings, *Benefits for Survivors of Retired Military Personnel.* 1980. Report No. 96-62. Ninety-sixth Congress, Second Session.

Holmes, R. A., Hillsman, T. C., Small, E. M., and Borthwick, R. B. 1978. Military retirement: The role of youth and vigor. In *Supplementary Papers of The President's Commission on Military Compensation,* Vol. 2. Washington, D. C.: U. S. Gov't. Printing Office.

Hook, C. R. 1948. *Advisory Commission on Service Pay of the Department of Defense.* Washington, D. C.: U. S. Gov't. Printing Office.

Inquiry Into Survivor Benefits. 1970. Report of Special Subcommittee on Survivor Benefits of The House Committee on Armed Services. Ninety-first Congress, Second Session.

Interagency Committee. 1971. *Report To The President on The Study of Uniformed Services Retirement and Survivor Benefits.* Washington, D. C.: U. S. Gov't. Printing Office.

Janowitz, M. 1960. *The Professional Soldier.* Glencoe, Ill.: The Free Press.

Kilpatrick, A. C. and Kilpatrick, E. G. 1979. Retirement from the military: Problems of adjustment. *Social Casework* 60:282-88.

Kuzmack, R. A. 1978. Deferred compensation and social security in the military retirement system. *Report by Math Tech to the President's Commission on Military Compensation.* Arlington, Va.

McCubbin, H. I., Dahl, B. B., and Hunter, E. J. 1976. *Families in the Military System.* Beverly Hills, Calif.: Sage Publications.

Maynard, C. and Blalock, A. 1977. The welfare state within the military. *Journal of Sociology and Social Welfare* 4:494-521.

McNeil, J. S. 1964. Adjustment of Retired Air Force Officers: Unpublished doctoral dissertation, University of Southern Calif.

McNeil, J. S. 1976. Individual and family problems related to retirement from the military service. In H. I. McCubbin, B. B. Dahl, and E. J. Hunter (eds.) *Families in the Military System.* Beverly Hills, Calif.: Sage Publications.

McNeil, J. S. and Giffen, M. B. 1965a. Military retirement: Some basic observations and concepts. *Journal of Aerospace Medicine* 36:25-29.

________. 1965b. The social impact of military retirement. *Social Casework* 46:203-7.

________. 1967. Military retirement: The retirement syndrome. *American Journal of Psychiatry* 123:848-54.

Military Compensation Task Force. 1976. Directorate of Human Resources Development, Office of the Deputy Chief of Staff for Personnel, Vol. I, U. S. Army.

Military Retiree Survey Report. 1978. Department of Defense. Washington, D. C.: Office of The Assistant Secretary of Defense for Military Personnel Policy.

Milowe, I. D. 1964. A study in role diffusion: The chief and the sergeant face retirement. *Mental Hygiene* 48:101-7.

Morse, D. W. and Gray, S. H. 1980. *Early Retirement, Boon or Bane?* Montclair, N. J.: Allanheld, Osmun Publishers.

Ogburn, B., Bellino, R., Williams, R., and Gordon, R. 1969. Problems of the military retiree. *The Journal of the Florida Medical Association* 50:245-48.

Parad, G. 1960. A framework for studying families in crisis. *Social Work.*

Parker, J. F., Jr., Christensen, D. G., and Every, M. G. 1978. A review of the youth and vigor concept and its importance in military occupations. In *Supplementary Papers of The President's Commission on Military Compensation.* Washington, D. C.: U. S. Gov't. Printing Office.

Platte, R. J. 1976. The second career: Perceived social mobility and adjustment among recent army retirees and wives of army retirees. In H. I. McCubbin, B. B. Dahl, and E. J. Hunter (eds.) *Families in the Military System.* Beverly Hills, Calif.: Sage Publications.

Reed, L. S. 1975. Military Maneuvers: *Analysis of the Interchange of Personnel Between Defense Contractors and the Development of Defense.* New York: Council on Economic Priorities.

Report of The President's Commission on Military Compensation. 1978. Washington, D. C.: U. S. Gov't Printing Office.

Report of The Subcommittee on Investigations of The House Committee on Post Office and Civil Service. 1977. Ninety-fifth Congress, First Session.

Report of The Subcommittee on Investigations of The House Committee on Post Office and Civil Service, *Dual Compensation Paid to Retired Uniformed Services Personnel.* 1978. Ninety-fifth Congress, Second Session.

Retirement Supplement, *Army Times,* July 12, 1982.

Sharp, L. M. and Biderman, A. D. 1966. *The Employment of Retired Military Personnel.* Washington, D. C.: Bureau of Social Science Research.

Taussig, J. K., Jr. 1981. A review of post-retirement employment restrictions. *The Retired Officer* 27, No. 1.

Tilove, Robert. 1976. *Public Employee Pension Funds.* New York: Columbia University Press.

Third Quadrennial Review of Military Compensation. 1976. Department of Defense. *Military Compensation Background Papers: Compensation Elements and Related Manpower Cost Items Their Purpose and Legislative Background,* Washington, D. C.: U. S. Gov't. Printing Office.

Title 30 United States Statute 1006, 1899.

Title 44 United States Statute 531, 1926.

Title 62 United States Statute 1081, 1948.

Title 63 United States Statute 802, 1949.

Title 27 United States Statute 348, 1982.

U. S. Air Force News for Retired Personnel, April, 1961.

U. S. Congress. 1861. *Statutes At Large.* Thirty-seventh Congress, First Session, Chapter 42, Section 15.

———. 1882. *Statutes At Large.* Forty-seventh Congress, First Session, Chapter 254.

———. 1935. *Statutes At Large.* Seventy-fourth Congress, First Session, Chapter 422.

University of Michigan Study. 1961. *A Study of The Military Retired System and Certain Related Subjects.* A Report to The Committee on Armed Services of the U. S. Senate.

Watson, J. H. 1963. *A Study of Social and Occupational Adjustment in Relation to Civilian and Military Identification of United States Air Force Officers.* Unpublished Ph.D. dissertation, University of Southern Mississippi.

West, B. S. 1980. Pre-retirement education: Planning the future with a new approach. *Occupational Health and Safety* 49:5.

Wolpert, D. S., Patrissi, G. A., and Littlepage, J. R. 1982. *A Survey of retirement plans and expectations.* Unpublished report.

INDEX

ABOUT THE AUTHORS

John S. McNeil, a retired Air Force Colonel, is currently Associate Professor at the Graduate School of Social Work, University of Texas at Arlington. He has published numerous articles in the field of military retirement.

Pedro J. Lecca is a Lt. Colonel, Army Reserve, and Professor at the Graduate School of Social Work, University of Texas at Arlington. He is coauthor of numerous titles in the field of health care.

Roosevelt Wright, Jr. is currently Associate Professor at the Graduate School of Social Work, University of Texas at Arlington. He is coauthor of *Transcultural Perspectives in the Human Services* and *Black Alcoholism.*

DATE DUE
